NATURAL REMEDIES FOR OVERCOMING DEPRESSION

A Comprehensive Guide to Herbal Remedies, Mind-Body Practices, and Holistic Approaches for Mental Well-being

ADOOH MARCEL

DEDICATION

This book is dedicated to God almighty and my entire family for their unwavering support, boundless encouragement, and profound love they have showered upon me throughout my life and in the course of writing this book. They are the beating heart of my existence, and I want the world to know just how profoundly I appreciate their presence in my journey. And I pray that the almighty God bless them all.

Copyright 2023 – Adooh Marcel

Table of Contents

INTRODUCTION

Millions of individuals worldwide suffer from depression, a complicated and widespread mental health illness. Characterized by persistent feelings of sadness, hopelessness, and a lack of interest or pleasure in daily activities, depression can have a profound impact on an individual's quality of life. While medical interventions such as antidepressant medications and therapy play a crucial role in treating depression, there is a growing interest in natural remedies as complementary approaches to support mental well-being.

This comprehensive guide aims to explore various natural remedies for overcoming depression, emphasizing holistic and lifestyle-based approaches. By addressing the interconnected facets of physical health, mental well-being, and social support, individuals may find additional tools to enhance their resilience and cope with depressive symptoms.

In the following sections, we will delve into the causes of depression, lifestyle changes that can positively influence mental health, herbal remedies with potential mood-boosting properties, mind-body practices that promote relaxation, holistic approaches like acupuncture and massage therapy, the importance of social connections, strategies for limiting negative influences, seeking professional guidance when necessary, and the ongoing self-care practices that contribute to long-term mental well-being.

It is essential to approach these natural remedies as part of a comprehensive and personalized mental health plan. Individuals experiencing depression should consult with healthcare professionals to determine the most appropriate and effective interventions for their unique circumstances. This guide serves as a resource for understanding and integrating natural remedies into a broader framework of mental health care.

CHAPTER ONE
CAUSES OF DEPRESSION

Depression is a multifaceted condition influenced by a combination of biological, psychological, and social factors. Understanding these causes is crucial for developing effective strategies for prevention and treatment. In this section, we explore the various contributors to depression:

BIOLOGICAL FACTORS

The development of depression is significantly influenced by biological variables. These factors involve the complex interplay of genetic, neurological, and hormonal elements. Understanding the biological basis of depression helps shed light on why certain individuals may be more predisposed to the condition. Here are key biological factors associated with depression:

1. **Genetic Factors:**
   - **Family History:** Individuals with a family history of depression are at a higher risk. There is evidence to suggest that genetic factors contribute to the heritability of depression.
   - **Gene Variants:** Specific genes and gene variations have been implicated in depression. These genes may influence neurotransmitter function, stress response, and brain structure.
2. **Neurotransmitter Imbalances:**
   - **Serotonin:** Changes in serotonin levels, a neurotransmitter associated with mood regulation have been linked to depression. Antidepressant medications often target the serotonin system.
   - **Dopamine and Norepinephrine:** Imbalances in these neurotransmitters, which are involved in reward, motivation, and alertness, can also contribute to depressive symptoms.

3. **Brain Structure and Function:**
    - **Hippocampus:** Changes in the size and function of the hippocampus, a brain region involved in memory and emotion regulation, have been observed in people with depression.
    - **Amygdala:** The amygdala, which plays a role in processing emotions, may be hyperactive in individuals with depression, contributing to heightened emotional responses.
    - **Prefrontal Cortex:** Changes in the prefrontal cortex, responsible for decision-making and emotional regulation, are associated with depressive symptoms.
4. **Hormonal Factors:**
    - **Endocrine System:** Hormones such as cortisol, the body's primary stress hormone, are often dysregulated in individuals with depression Prolonged rise of cortisol levels can be caused by chronic stress.
    - **Thyroid Function:** Abnormalities in thyroid function, including hypothyroidism, can contribute to depressive symptoms.
5. **Inflammatory Processes:**
    - **Inflammation:** Elevated levels of inflammatory markers have been found in some individuals with depression. Chronic inflammation may influence the development and persistence of depressive symptoms.
6. **Neuroplasticity:**
    - **Brain Changes:** Depression is associated with alterations in neuroplasticity, the brain's ability to adapt and reorganize itself. Changes in synaptic connections and neural circuits may contribute to the symptoms of depression.

It's important to note that while these biological factors are associated with depression, they interact with environmental and psychosocial factors, contributing to the complexity of the condition. Additionally, not everyone with a genetic predisposition or neurological changes will necessarily develop depression, as environmental factors also play a crucial role in its onset and course. A holistic understanding that considers both biological and environmental factors is crucial for effectively addressing and treating depression.

PSYCHOLOGICAL FACTORS

Psychological factors play a crucial role in the development, maintenance, and treatment of depression. These factors involve aspects of an individual's thoughts, emotions, and behavior. Understanding the psychological dimensions of depression helps inform therapeutic approaches and interventions. Here are key psychological factors associated with depression:

1. **Cognitive Factors:**
    - **Cognitive Distortions:** Distorted thought patterns, such as negative thinking, catastrophizing, and overgeneralization, can contribute to the development and maintenance of depressive symptoms.
    - **Negative Self-Perception:** Low self-esteem and a negative self-image are common features of depression. Individuals may perceive themselves as unworthy or incapable.
2. **Stressful Life Events:**
    - **Significant Life Transitions:** Severe or extremely stressful life events, such the death of a loved one, divorce, losing a job, or facing financial hardships, can cause or worsen depression.
    - **Chronic Stress:** Prolonged exposure to chronic stressors, whether interpersonal, work-related, or environmental, can contribute to the development of depression.
3. **Personality Factors:**
    - **Neuroticism:** Individuals with high levels of neuroticism, characterized by emotional instability and a tendency to experience negative emotions, may be more susceptible to depression.
    - **Perfectionism:** Excessive perfectionism, setting unrealistically high standards for oneself, can contribute to chronic stress and a vulnerability to depression.
4. **Coping Strategies:**

- **Maladaptive Coping:** Ineffective coping mechanisms, such as avoidance, substance abuse, or self-isolation, can contribute to the escalation of depressive symptoms.
- **Rumination:** Excessive rumination, or dwelling on negative thoughts and feelings, can prolong and intensify depressive episodes.

5. **Attachment Style:**
   - **Insecure Attachments:** Early experiences with caregivers can influence attachment styles. Insecure attachments, characterized by a lack of emotional security and trust, may contribute to vulnerability to depression.

6. **Learned Helplessness:**
   - **Learned Helplessness Theory:** According to this theory, individuals who perceive events as beyond their control and believe they cannot influence outcomes may develop a sense of helplessness, which is associated with depression.

7. **Interpersonal Relationships:**
   - **Social Isolation:** Depression may be exacerbated by feelings of social isolation and a lack of support from others. Protective elements include supportive partnerships and positive social ties.
   - **Interpersonal Conflict:** Strained relationships or conflict within interpersonal relationships can contribute to and exacerbate depressive symptoms.

8. **Coping Skills and Resilience:**
   - **Adaptive Coping:** Developing effective coping skills, problem-solving abilities, and resilience can enhance an individual's capacity to manage stress and reduce the risk of depression.

Understanding these psychological factors is essential for developing targeted interventions in the treatment of depression. Cognitive-behavioral therapy (CBT), for example, is an evidence-based therapeutic approach that addresses maladaptive thought patterns and behaviors associated with depression. Additionally, improving coping skills, fostering positive social connections, and addressing underlying stressors are integral components of comprehensive treatment plans for depression.

SOCIAL FACTORS

Social factors play a significant role in the development, expression, and management of depression. These factors involve an individual's interactions with their social environment, including relationships, societal influences, and cultural contexts. Understanding the social dimensions of depression is crucial for a comprehensive perspective on this complex mental health condition. Here are key social factors associated with depression:

1. **Social Support:**
   - **Lack of Social Support:** A lack of supportive relationships and social isolation are risk factors for depression. Positive social interactions and a strong support system can act as protective factors against the onset and severity of depressive symptoms.
2. **Interpersonal Relationships:**
   - **Conflict and Strain:** Conflict within relationships, whether with family members, friends, or romantic partners, can contribute to the development and exacerbation of depressive symptoms.
   - **Loss and Grief:** The loss of a loved one through death, separation, or other forms of loss can trigger or intensify depressive episodes.
3. **Family Dynamics:**
   - **Family History:** A family history of depression or mental health issues can increase an individual's vulnerability to the condition. Family dynamics and the quality of family relationships can impact mental health.

4. **Cultural and Societal Norms:**
   - **Stigma:** Societal stigma surrounding mental health issues, including depression, may discourage individuals from seeking help and contribute to feelings of shame or isolation.
   - **Cultural Influences:** Cultural attitudes and expectations regarding mental health, expressions of emotion, and help-

seeking behavior can shape the way depression is experienced and addressed.

5. **Economic Factors:**
   - **Financial Stress:** Economic challenges, unemployment, or financial instability can contribute to chronic stress and increase the risk of depression.
   - **Socioeconomic Status:** Disparities in socioeconomic status can impact access to resources, educational opportunities, and healthcare, influencing mental health outcomes.

6. **Life Transitions:**
   - **Major Life Changes:** Events such as job loss, relocation, divorce, or retirement can be sources of stress and may contribute to the development of depression.
   - **Transition to Parenthood:** Postpartum depression is a particular type of depression that can arise from a mix of hormonal, psychological, and social causes following childbirth.

7. **Social Comparison:**
   - **Social Media Influence:** Excessive use of social media, where individuals often present curated and idealized versions of their lives, can contribute to social comparison and feelings of inadequacy, potentially exacerbating depressive symptoms.

8. **Discrimination and Marginalization:**
   - **Systemic Discrimination:** Experiences of discrimination based on factors such as race, gender, sexual orientation, or other identity-related factors can contribute to stress and increase vulnerability to depression.

Addressing social factors in the context of depression often involves a multi-faceted approach. Interventions may include building social support networks, improving communication skills, addressing systemic issues related to discrimination, and promoting awareness and understanding of mental health within communities. Additionally, creating supportive environments and reducing societal stigma can contribute to a more positive and inclusive approach to mental health.

CHAPTER TWO
LIFESTYLE CHANGES

Lifestyle changes can have a significant impact on mental health, including the prevention and management of depression. While lifestyle adjustments may not replace professional treatment for individuals with clinical depression, they can complement therapeutic interventions and contribute to overall well-being. Here are some lifestyle changes that may be beneficial:

1. **Regular Exercise:**
   - **Benefits:** Exercise is associated with the release of neurotransmitters such as endorphins, which can improve mood. It also reduces stress hormones and promotes better sleep.
   - **Recommendations:** Aim for at least 150 minutes of moderate-intensity exercise per week, such as brisk walking, jogging, or cycling.
2. **Healthy Diet:**
   - **Nutrient-Rich Foods:** Consuming a diet rich in fruits, vegetables, whole grains, lean proteins, and omega-3 fatty acids supports brain health and may have positive effects on mood.
   - **Limiting Sugar and Processed Foods:** High-sugar and processed foods can contribute to energy fluctuations and impact mood.
3. **Adequate Sleep:**
   - **Importance of Sleep:** Sleep plays a crucial role in mood regulation and overall mental health. Establishing a regular sleep routine and ensuring adequate sleep duration are essential.
   - **Sleep Hygiene Practices:** Create a comfortable sleep environment, limit screen time before bedtime, and avoid caffeine close to bedtime.

4. **Stress Management:**
   - **Mindfulness and Relaxation Techniques:** Practices such as meditation, deep breathing exercises, and yoga can help manage stress and promote emotional well-being.
   - **Time management:** Stress and feelings of overburden can be lessened by planning chores and establishing reasonable objectives.
5. **Social Connections:**
   - **Quality Relationships:** Nurturing positive relationships and maintaining a social support network are crucial for emotional well-being.
   - **Joining Groups or Clubs:** Participating in activities or groups that align with personal interests can provide opportunities to connect with others.
6. **Limiting Alcohol and Substance Use:**
   - **Impact on Mental Health:** Excessive alcohol and substance use can contribute to or exacerbate depressive symptoms. Moderation or abstinence may be advisable.
   - **Seeking Help:** If substance use becomes a concern, seeking professional help is important.
7. **Engaging in Hobbies and Activities:**
   - **Pleasurable Activities:** Participating in activities that bring joy and a sense of accomplishment can positively impact mood.
   - **Setting Realistic Goals:** Establishing achievable goals and celebrating small successes can contribute to a sense of purpose.
8. **Cognitive-Behavioral Techniques:**
   - **Identifying and Challenging Negative Thoughts:** Cognitive-behavioral techniques involve recognizing and changing negative thought patterns that contribute to depressive feelings.
   - **Goal Setting:** Setting and working towards realistic and meaningful goals can provide a sense of purpose and accomplishment.

9. **Professional Support:**
    - **Therapy and Counseling:** Seeking support from mental health professionals, such as therapists or counselors, can provide coping strategies, insights, and a safe space to explore emotions.
    - **Medication Management:** For individuals with clinical depression, medication prescribed by a healthcare professional may be an important component of treatment.

It's essential to approach lifestyle changes gradually and seek professional guidance, especially for those experiencing severe or persistent depressive symptoms. Tailoring these changes to individual preferences and needs can enhance their effectiveness in promoting mental health and well-being.

IMPORTANCE OF A BALANCED DIET

Maintaining a balanced diet is crucial for overall health and well-being, and it plays a significant role in supporting both physical and mental health. Here are some key reasons why a balanced diet is important:

1. **Nutrient Intake:**
    - **Essential Nutrients:** A balanced diet provides essential nutrients, including vitamins, minerals, proteins, carbohydrates, and fats, that the body needs for optimal functioning.
    - **Micronutrients:** Adequate intake of micronutrients, such as vitamins and minerals, supports various physiological processes, including immune function, energy production, and brain health.
2. **Energy Levels:**
    - **Stable Blood Sugar:** A balanced diet helps maintain stable blood sugar levels, preventing energy crashes and fatigue. Consuming a mix of complex carbohydrates, proteins, and healthy fats contributes to sustained energy throughout the day.

3. **Weight Management:**
   - **Caloric Balance:** A balanced diet promotes a healthy balance between calorie intake and expenditure, which is essential for weight management.
   - **Nutrient Density:** Choosing nutrient-dense foods over calorie-dense, processed foods supports weight management by providing essential nutrients without excessive calories.
4. **Digestive Health:**
   - **Fiber Intake:** A diet rich in fruits, vegetables, and whole grains provides fiber, which supports digestive health by promoting regular bowel movements and preventing constipation.
   - **Gut Microbiota:** Certain foods, like probiotics found in fermented foods, can contribute to a healthy balance of gut microbiota, which is linked to overall well-being.
5. **Heart Health:**
   - **Healthy Fats:** Including sources of healthy fats, such as omega-3 fatty acids found in fish and flaxseeds can help maintain cardiovascular health by reducing cholesterol levels and supporting proper heart function.
6. **Bone Health:**
   - **Calcium and Vitamin D:** A balanced diet with sufficient calcium and vitamin D is important for maintaining bone health and preventing conditions like osteoporosis.
7. **Brain Function:**
   - **Nutrient Support:** Proper nutrition is crucial for brain function, and certain nutrients play a role in cognitive function and mood regulation. For example, omega-3 fatty acids are associated with brain health.
8. **Mood and Mental Health:**
   - **Serotonin Production:** Adequate intake of nutrients like tryptophan, found in certain foods, supports the production of serotonin, a neurotransmitter associated with mood regulation.
   - **Blood Sugar Stability:** Fluctuations in blood sugar levels, which can result from an imbalanced diet, may impact mood and contribute to symptoms of anxiety and irritability.

9. **Disease Prevention:**
    - **Reducing Risk Factors:** A balanced diet can help reduce the risk of chronic diseases such as diabetes, cardiovascular diseases, and certain cancers by providing the necessary nutrients for optimal health.
10. **Long-Term Well-Being:**
    - **Healthy Aging:** A balanced diet contributes to overall well-being and supports healthy aging by providing the nutrients needed to maintain bodily functions and prevent age-related diseases.

It's important to note that individual dietary needs may vary based on factors such as age, gender, activity level, and underlying health conditions. Consulting with a healthcare professional or a registered dietitian can help tailor dietary recommendations to individual needs and goals. Additionally, making sustainable and realistic changes to dietary habits over time is key to reaping the long-term benefits of a balanced diet.

REGULAR EXERCISE AND ITS IMPACT

Regular exercise has a profound impact on overall health and well-being, affecting various aspects of physical, mental, and emotional health. Incorporating regular physical activity into one's routine has numerous benefits, and these effects extend beyond just physical fitness. Here are some key impacts of regular exercise:

PHYSICAL HEALTH BENEFITS:

1. **Cardiovascular Health:**
    - Regular exercise helps improve cardiovascular health by strengthening the heart and improving blood circulation.
    - It lowers blood pressure and reduces the risk of heart diseases and stroke.
2. **Weight Management:**
    - Physical activity is crucial for maintaining a healthy weight by burning calories and promoting the balance between energy intake and expenditure.

3. **Muscle Strength and Flexibility:**
   - Exercise contributes to the development of muscle strength and enhances flexibility, improving overall physical function.
   - Resistance training, in particular, helps build and maintain muscle mass.
4. **Bone Health:**

- Weight-bearing activities lower the risk of osteoporosis and increase bone density, such as jogging, weightlifting, and walking.

5. **Improved Immune Function:**
   - Regular exercise boosts the immune system, making the body more resilient to infections and illnesses.
6. **Joint Health:**
   - Physical activity helps maintain joint health by promoting lubrication and preventing stiffness.

MENTAL AND EMOTIONAL HEALTH BENEFITS:

1. **Mood Enhancement:**
   - Exercise stimulates the release of endorphins, the body's natural mood lifters, leading to improved mood and reduced feelings of stress and anxiety.
2. **Stress Reduction:**
   - Physical activity acts as a stress reliever by reducing levels of stress hormones like cortisol.
   - It provides a healthy outlet for managing and coping with daily stressors.
3. **Improved Sleep:**
   - Regular exercise can contribute to better sleep quality and may help alleviate symptoms of insomnia.
4. **Cognitive Function:**
   - Exercise has positive effects on cognitive function, including memory, attention, and problem-solving skills.
   - It could lessen the chance of neurodegenerative illnesses and cognitive deterioration.

5. **Increased Energy Levels:**
   - Despite expending energy during exercise, individuals often report increased energy levels throughout the day.

SOCIAL AND EMOTIONAL BENEFITS:

1. **Social Interaction:**
   - Group activities, team sports, or exercise classes provide opportunities for social interaction and the development of social support networks.
2. **Improved Self-Esteem:**
   - Regular physical activity is associated with improved self-esteem and body image, fostering a positive self-perception.
3. **Sense of Achievement:**
   - Setting and achieving fitness goals, whether small or large, contributes to a sense of accomplishment and self-efficacy.
4. **Enhanced Social Well-Being:**
   - Participation in community-based or team sports fosters a sense of belonging and community, promoting overall social well-being.

LONG-TERM HEALTH BENEFITS:

1. **Disease Prevention:**
   - Regular exercise is linked to a lower risk of chronic diseases such as type 2 diabetes, certain cancers, and metabolic syndrome.
2. **Increased Lifespan:**
   - Engaging in regular physical activity is associated with a longer and healthier lifespan.

It's important to note that the type and intensity of exercise can vary based on individual fitness levels, preferences, and health conditions. Before starting a new exercise program, it's advisable to consult with a healthcare professional, especially for individuals with pre-existing health conditions or concerns. Incorporating a variety of activities, including aerobic exercises, strength training, and flexibility exercises, can maximize the overall health benefits of regular physical activity.

SUFFICIENT SLEEP FOR MENTAL HEALTH

Sufficient sleep is crucial for maintaining good mental health and overall well-being. The relationship between sleep and mental health is bidirectional, meaning that both the quantity and quality of sleep can influence mental health, and mental health can affect sleep patterns. Here are several reasons why sufficient sleep is essential for mental health:

1. Emotional Regulation:

- **Stabilizing Mood:** Sleep plays a vital role in regulating emotions and mood. Anger, mood swings, and an increased responsiveness to emotions are all associated with sleep deprivation.

2. Cognitive Function:

- **Attention and Concentration:** Adequate sleep supports cognitive functions such as attention, concentration, and problem-solving abilities. Sleep deprivation can impair these functions and lead to difficulties in daily tasks.

3. Stress Reduction:

- **Cortisol Regulation:** Sleep helps regulate the body's stress hormone, cortisol. Chronic sleep deprivation can contribute to elevated cortisol levels, increasing stress and anxiety.

4. Memory Consolidation:

- **Learning and Memory:** Sleep is crucial for memory consolidation, the process by which the brain strengthens and stabilizes newly acquired information. Sufficient sleep enhances learning and memory.

5. Psychiatric Disorders:

- **Risk Reduction:** Insufficient sleep has been linked to an increased risk of developing mental health disorders, including depression, anxiety, and bipolar disorder.
- **Symptom Aggravation:** For individuals with existing mental health conditions, lack of sleep can exacerbate symptoms and make it more challenging to manage their condition.

6. Resilience to Stress:

- **Coping Mechanisms:** A well-rested mind is better equipped to cope with stressors, and individuals tend to be more resilient in the face of challenges when they've had sufficient sleep.

7. Regulation of Neurotransmitters:

- **Serotonin and Dopamine:** Sleep influences the regulation of neurotransmitters like serotonin and dopamine, which are essential for mood regulation. Disruptions in sleep patterns can impact these neurotransmitters.

8. Physical Health:

- **Immune System Support:** Quality sleep supports a healthy immune system, and a strong immune system is linked to better mental health.
- **Inflammation Reduction:** Chronic sleep deprivation may contribute to increased inflammation, which is associated with various mental health disorders.

9. Daytime Functioning:

- **Productivity and Alertness:** A good night's sleep enhances daytime alertness, productivity, and overall functioning.

10. Hormonal Regulation:

- **Melatonin Production:** Sleep is essential for the production of melatonin, a hormone that regulates the sleep-wake cycle. Disruptions in sleep can impact melatonin levels.

TIPS FOR IMPROVING SLEEP FOR BETTER MENTAL HEALTH:

- **Create a Regular Sleep Schedule:** Even on weekends, go to bed and wake up at the same time every day.
- **Establish a Calm Bedtime Routine:** Before going to bed, perform some soothing activities to let your body know it's time to unwind.

- **Create a Comfortable Sleep Environment:** Keep your bedroom dark, quiet, and at a comfortable temperature.
- **Limit Stimulants:** Steer clear of coffee and nicotine, especially in the few hours before bed.
- **Limit Screen Time:** Reduce exposure to screens (phones, computers, TVs) at least an hour before bedtime, as the blue light emitted can interfere with melatonin production.

Prioritizing sufficient, good-quality sleep is an essential component of a holistic approach to mental health and well-being. Individuals experiencing persistent sleep difficulties or significant changes in sleep patterns should consider consulting with a healthcare professional for further evaluation and guidance.

CHAPTER THREE
HERBAL REMEDIES

Herbal remedies, derived from plants and plant extracts, have been used for centuries in various cultures for medicinal purposes. While herbal remedies are often perceived as natural and may offer certain benefits, it's important to approach them with caution. The efficacy and safety of herbal remedies can vary, and their use should be discussed with a healthcare professional, especially if someone is already taking medications or has underlying health conditions. Here are some herbal remedies that are commonly associated with potential mental health benefits:

ST. JOHN'S WORT: NATURE'S ANTIDEPRESSANT

St. John's Wort (Hypericum perforatum) is a flowering plant with yellow petals that has been traditionally used for its potential medicinal properties, particularly in addressing symptoms of depression. It is often referred to as "nature's antidepressant" due to its historical use for mood-related concerns. Here are key points about St. John's Wort:

1. Traditional Use:

- St. John's Wort has a long history of use in traditional medicine, particularly in European folk medicine.
- Ancient Greek and Roman physicians used it to treat various ailments, including mood disorders.

2. Active Compounds:

- Hypericin and hyperforin are two of the active compounds believed to contribute to the plant's potential antidepressant effects.
- These compounds are thought to influence neurotransmitters in the brain, including serotonin, dopamine, and norepinephrine.

3. Antidepressant Effects:

- St. John's Wort has been studied for its potential in treating mild to moderate depression.
- Some studies suggest that it may be as effective as certain conventional antidepressants, particularly for mild cases.

4. Mechanism of Action:

- The exact mechanism of St. John's Wort's antidepressant action is not fully understood.
- It is believed to modulate the levels of neurotransmitters in the brain, similar to the action of some prescription antidepressants.

5. Other Potential Benefits:

- St. John's Wort has been explored for other potential benefits, including its anti-inflammatory, antioxidant, and antiviral properties.
- Some studies suggest potential benefits for conditions such as anxiety and premenstrual syndrome (PMS).

6. Caution and Considerations:

- **Interactions:** St. John's Wort can interact with a variety of medications, including certain antidepressants, birth control pills, and anticoagulants. It can reduce the effectiveness of these medications.
- **Side Effects:** While generally considered safe for short-term use, St. John's Wort may cause side effects such as gastrointestinal upset, fatigue, and sensitivity to sunlight.
- **Quality and Dosage:** The quality of St. John's Wort supplements can vary, and dosage recommendations may differ. Standardization of the product is important for consistency.

7. Consultation with Healthcare Professionals:

- Individuals considering St. John's Wort for depression or other mental health concerns should consult with a healthcare professional.
- It is essential to inform healthcare providers about all medications, including herbal supplements, to avoid potential interactions.

8. Regulatory Status:

- St. John's Wort is available over the counter in many countries as a dietary supplement.
- Regulatory standards for herbal supplements vary, and it's important to choose products from reputable manufacturers.

9. Research Limitations:

- While some studies suggest benefits, the overall body of research on St. John's Wort is not as extensive as that for certain prescription antidepressants.
- Further research is needed to establish its efficacy, optimal dosage, and long-term safety.

It's crucial to approach the use of St. John's Wort with caution and under the guidance of a healthcare professional, especially for individuals with depression or those taking prescription medications. While some people may find it beneficial, it's not a substitute for professional medical advice and treatment. Always consult with a healthcare provider before starting any new supplement or making significant changes to your health regimen.

LAVENDER OIL FOR RELAXATION

Lavender oil, derived from the lavender plant (Lavandula), is renowned for its pleasant aroma and has been used for centuries for various purposes, including relaxation and stress relief. Here are key points regarding the use of lavender oil for relaxation:

1. Aromatherapy:

- **Primary Use:** Lavender oil is commonly used in aromatherapy, a practice that involves inhaling the fragrance of essential oils to promote well-being.
- **Calming Effect:** The aroma of lavender is often associated with relaxation and is believed to have calming effects on the nervous system.

2. Mechanism of Action:

- **Linalool and Linalyl Acetate:** Lavender oil contains compounds such as linalool and linalyl acetate, which are thought to contribute to its relaxing properties.
- **Impact on Neurotransmitters:** The aroma of lavender may influence neurotransmitters such as serotonin, promoting a sense of calm.

3. Stress Reduction:

- **Cortisol Levels:** Some studies suggest that exposure to lavender scent may help reduce cortisol levels, the hormone associated with stress.
- **Anxiety Reduction:** Lavender oil has been studied for its potential in reducing symptoms of anxiety and promoting relaxation.

4. Sleep Aid:

- **Improving Sleep Quality:** Lavender oil is often used to promote better sleep. It's relaxing effects may help individuals unwind and improve the overall quality of sleep.
- **Insomnia:** It has been explored as a complementary approach for managing symptoms of insomnia.

5. Application Methods:

- **Diffusion:** Adding a few drops of lavender oil to a diffuser can disperse the aroma throughout a room.
- **Topical Application:** Some people choose to dilute lavender oil with a carrier oil and apply it topically, such as on the wrists or temples.
- **Bathing:** Adding a few drops of lavender oil to a warm bath can create a soothing experience.

6. Caution and Considerations:

- **Skin Sensitivity:** While lavender oil is generally considered safe, some individuals may experience skin sensitivity or irritation. Before using it on more exposed skin, it is best to conduct a patch test.
- **Ingestion:** Ingesting essential oils is not recommended without guidance from a qualified healthcare professional.

7. Individual Variability:

- **Personal Preferences:** Responses to aromatherapy, including lavender oil, can vary among individuals. Some people find the scent highly relaxing, while others may not have the same response.

8. Complementary Approach:

- **Supportive, Not a Replacement:** Lavender oil is often used as a complementary approach to relaxation and stress reduction. It should not replace professional mental health interventions for individuals dealing with significant stress, anxiety, or other mental health concerns.

9. Quality Matters:

- **Choosing a Quality Product:** When selecting lavender oil, it's important to choose a high-quality, pure essential oil to ensure its efficacy and safety.

10. Professional Guidance:

- **Consultation with Healthcare Providers:** Individuals with pre-existing health conditions or those pregnant should consult with a healthcare professional before using essential oils, including lavender oil.

While many people find lavender oil to be a soothing and pleasant addition to their relaxation routines, it's essential to approach its use with individual considerations in mind. If someone is dealing with persistent stress, anxiety, or sleep disturbances, it's advisable to seek guidance from a healthcare professional for a comprehensive and personalized approach to mental well-being.

VALERIAN ROOT AND ITS CALMING EFFECTS

Valerian root (Valeriana officinalis) is an herb that has been traditionally used for its potential calming and sedative effects. Here are key points regarding valerian root and its calming properties:

1. Traditional Use:

- Valerian root has a long history of use in traditional medicine, dating back to ancient Greece and Rome.
- It gained popularity for its reported calming and sedative properties.

2. Active Compounds:

- Valerian root contains various compounds, including valerenic acid, which is believed to contribute to its potential sedative effects.

- Some studies suggest that valerian may interact with gamma-aminobutyric acid (GABA) receptors in the brain, similar to the action of certain anti-anxiety medications.

3. Anxiolytic Effects:

- Valerian root has been studied for its potential anxiolytic (anxiety-reducing) effects.
- Some users report feeling a sense of calmness and relaxation after consuming valerian root.

4. Sleep Aid:

- Valerian root is a popular natural sleep aid that may shorten the time it takes to fall asleep and enhance the quality of sleep.

5. Mechanism of Action:

- The exact mechanism by which valerian root exerts its calming effects is not fully understood.
- It is thought to enhance the inhibitory neurotransmitter GABA, leading to a calming impact on the central nervous system.

6. Usage Forms:

- Valerian root is available in various forms, including tea, capsules, and liquid extracts.
- Valerian root tea is a popular choice for those seeking a natural way to promote relaxation.

7. Caution and Considerations:

- Responses to valerian root can vary among individuals. Some people could noticeably feel calmer, but others might not.

- Valerian may interact with certain medications, including sedatives and medications that affect the central nervous system. Consultation with a healthcare provider is advised, especially if taking other medications.
- Pregnant or breastfeeding individuals should consult with a healthcare professional before using valerian root.

8. Quality Matters:

- Choosing a reputable product is important when selecting valerian root supplements. Ensure that the product is from a trustworthy manufacturer to guarantee quality and potency.

9. Short-Term Use:

- Valerian root is generally considered safe for short-term use.
- Limited evidence is available on its long-term safety, so extended use should be approached with caution.

10. Consultation with Healthcare Professionals:

- Individuals with pre-existing health conditions or those taking medications should consult with a healthcare professional before using valerian root for its calming effects.

11. Individual Variability:

- As with many herbal remedies, individual responses can vary. Some individuals may find valerian root highly effective for relaxation, while others may not experience the same benefits.

Valerian root is a widely used herbal remedy for promoting relaxation and improving sleep. While it is generally considered safe for short-term use, it's important to approach its use with caution, especially for individuals with underlying health conditions or those taking medications. Consulting with a healthcare professional can provide personalized guidance based on individual health needs.

CHAPTER FOUR
MIND-BODY PRACTICES

Mind-body practices involve techniques that integrate the mind and body to enhance health and well-being. These practices recognize the intricate connection between mental and physical health, emphasizing the influence of thoughts, emotions, and behaviors on overall wellness. Here are some popular mind-body practices:

YOGA FOR MENTAL WELL-BEING

Yoga is a mind-body practice that has been widely recognized for its positive impact on mental well-being. The integration of physical postures, breath control, meditation, and ethical principles makes yoga a holistic approach to promoting mental health. Here are several ways in which yoga contributes to mental well-being:

1. Stress Reduction:

- **Breath Awareness:** Yoga emphasizes conscious breathing (pranayama), which can activate the relaxation response and reduce the physiological effects of stress.
- **Mindfulness:** The practice of mindfulness in yoga encourages present-moment awareness, helping individuals let go of stressors from the past and worries about the future.

2. Anxiety Management:

- **GABA Production:** Some studies suggest that yoga may increase the production of gamma-aminobutyric acid (GABA), a neurotransmitter associated with reducing anxiety.
- **Mind-Body Connection:** The mind-body connection in yoga promotes a sense of grounding and calmness, which can be beneficial for managing anxiety.

3. Improved Mood:

- **Endorphin Release:** Physical activity in yoga, even in its gentler forms, can stimulate the release of endorphins, the body's natural mood enhancers.
- **Balancing Energy:** Yoga aims to balance the body's energy centers, contributing to emotional equilibrium.

4. Enhanced Emotional Regulation:

- **Mindfulness Practices:** Yoga often incorporates mindfulness techniques that cultivate awareness of thoughts and emotions without judgment. Better control over emotions may result from this.
- **Self-Reflection:** The reflective aspects of yoga encourage individuals to explore their inner experiences and develop a compassionate understanding of their emotions.

5. Cognitive Benefits:

- **Focus and Concentration:** The practice of holding yoga poses (asanas) and engaging in meditation enhances concentration and mental clarity.
- **Brain Plasticity:** Some research suggests that yoga may have positive effects on brain plasticity, potentially contributing to cognitive resilience.

6. Improved Sleep:

- **Relaxation Response:** The calming effects of yoga, particularly when practiced in the evening, can contribute to better sleep quality.
- **Reduction in Insomnia:** Yoga has been studied as a complementary approach to managing insomnia and improving sleep duration.

7. Social Connection:

- **Group Classes:** Participating in group yoga classes provides a sense of community and social connection, which is important for mental well-being.
- **Shared Experience:** The shared experience of practicing yoga with others can foster a supportive environment.

8. Mind-Body Awareness:

- **Body Scan:** Yoga encourages practitioners to pay attention to physical sensations and the present moment, promoting a deeper connection between the mind and body.
- **Acceptance:** Emphasizing self-acceptance and non-judgment, yoga helps individuals become more attuned to their bodies and emotions.

9. Coping with Trauma:

- **Trauma-Informed Yoga:** Specially adapted yoga practices, known as trauma-informed yoga, are designed to create a safe and supportive environment for individuals dealing with trauma.

10. Personal Empowerment:

- **Self-Efficacy:** As individuals progress in their yoga practice, they often experience increased self-efficacy and a sense of personal empowerment.
- **Resilience Building:** Yoga encourages the development of resilience in facing life's challenges.

TIPS FOR INCORPORATING YOGA FOR MENTAL WELL-BEING:

- **Start Slowly:** Begin with gentler yoga practices, especially if you are new to yoga.
- **Consistency:** Regular practice, even for shorter durations, can yield benefits over time.

- **Mindful Movement:** Focus on the present moment during yoga sessions, paying attention to breath and sensations.
- **Adapt to Your Needs:** Modify poses to suit your body and comfort level.
- **Seek Professional Guidance:** If dealing with specific mental health concerns, consider practicing yoga under the guidance of a certified instructor or mental health professional.

Yoga is a versatile practice that can be adapted to various needs and preferences. Whether practiced in a class setting or at home, the mindful and intentional nature of yoga makes it a valuable tool for promoting mental well-being. If you have specific mental health concerns, it's advisable to consult with a healthcare professional for personalized guidance and support.

MEDITATION TECHNIQUES

Meditation is a practice that involves focusing the mind and cultivating a state of heightened awareness, relaxation, and mental clarity. There are various meditation techniques, each with its own approach and benefits. Here are some common meditation techniques:

1. Mindfulness Meditation:

- **Overview:** Mindfulness meditation involves paying attention to the present moment without judgment. It often centers on the breath, sensations in the body, or the environment.
- **Practice:**
    - Find a quiet space and sit or lie down comfortably.
    - Focus on your breath, sensations, or an anchor point.
    - When distractions arise, gently bring your attention back to the present moment.

2. Loving-Kindness Meditation (Metta):

- **Overview:** Metta meditation focuses on cultivating feelings of love and compassion, both for oneself and others.

- **Practice:**
    - Start by extending love and kindness to yourself.
    - Gradually expand to loved ones, acquaintances, and even those you may find challenging.
    - Repeat phrases such as "May I/you be happy, may I/you be healthy" to foster positive intentions.

3. Body Scan Meditation:

- **Overview:** Body scan meditation involves bringing awareness to different parts of the body, progressively moving from head to toe or vice versa.
- **Practice:**
    - Begin by focusing on sensations in one part of the body.
    - Slowly move your attention through each body part, noticing any tension or sensations.
    - This practice enhances body awareness and relaxation.

4. Transcendental Meditation (TM):

- **Overview:** TM is a mantra meditation technique where practitioners repeat a specific sound or mantra silently.
- **Practice:**
    - Sit comfortably with eyes closed.
    - Repeat your chosen mantra silently.
    - If distractions arise, gently return to the mantra.

5. Zen Meditation (Zazen):

- **Overview:** Zazen, a form of seated meditation in Zen Buddhism, emphasizes mindful breathing and maintaining a still, focused posture.
- **Practice:**
    - Sit in a stable and comfortable position.
    - Focus on your breath or an aspect of your experience.
    - Allow thoughts to come and go without attachment.

6. Guided Meditation:

- **Overview:** Guided meditation involves following the verbal guidance of a teacher or recorded audio to lead you through a specific experience or visualization.
- **Practice:**
    - Listen to the guided instructions, which may involve imagery, relaxation, or mindfulness.
    - Guided meditations are suitable for beginners and those seeking specific outcomes.

7. Breath Awareness Meditation:

- **Overview:** This simple yet powerful meditation involves focusing on the breath to cultivate mindfulness and concentration.
- **Practice:**
    - Sit in a comfortable position and bring attention to the breath.
    - Observe the natural inhalation and exhalation.
    - Redirect the mind to the breath whenever it wanders.

8. Mantra Meditation:

- **Overview:** Mantra meditation involves repeating a word, sound, or phrase (mantra) to enhance concentration and create a meditative state.
- **Practice:**
    - Choose a mantra or receive one from a teacher.
    - Repeat the mantra silently or aloud with focused attention.
    - Allow the mantra to become a focal point for meditation.

9. Walking Meditation:

- **Overview:** Walking meditation combines mindfulness with walking, encouraging awareness of each step and the surrounding environment.
- **Practice:**
    - Walk slowly and deliberately, paying attention to each step.

- Maintain awareness of your body movements and breath.
- This practice can be done indoors or outdoors.

10. Body-Mind Connection Meditation:

- **Overview:** This type of meditation emphasizes the connection between the mind and body, fostering awareness of sensations, thoughts, and emotions.
- **Practice:**
    - Sit comfortably and bring attention to bodily sensations.
    - Observe thoughts and emotions without judgment.
    - Cultivate a sense of curiosity and non-reactivity.

TIPS FOR MEDITATION PRACTICE:

- **Consistency:** Establish a regular meditation routine to experience cumulative benefits.
- **Start Small:** Begin with shorter sessions and gradually extend the duration as you become more comfortable.
- **Comfortable Posture:** Sit or lie down in a comfortable position that allows alertness without strain.
- **Non-Judgmental Awareness:** Approach meditation with an open and non-judgmental mindset, acknowledging thoughts without criticism.
- **Guidance:** Beginners may benefit from guided meditations or attending meditation classes.
- **Patience:** Meditation is a skill that develops over time. Be patient with yourself as you explore different techniques.

Choose a meditation technique that resonates with you and aligns with your goals, whether it's cultivating mindfulness, reducing stress, or fostering a greater sense of well-being. Experiment with different practices to discover what works best for your unique preferences and needs.

DEEP BREATHING EXERCISES

Deep breathing exercises are a simple yet effective way to promote relaxation, reduce stress, and enhance overall well-being. These exercises typically involve slow, deliberate breathing patterns to activate the body's relaxation response. Here are several deep breathing techniques that you can try:

1. Diaphragmatic Breathing (Abdominal or Belly Breathing):

- **How to Practice:**
    - Sit or lie down comfortably.
    - Grasp your belly with one hand and your chest with the other.
    - Breathe in deeply and slowly through your nose, letting your stomach grow.
    - As you gently release the breath through your mouth, feel your stomach compress.
    - Repeat for several breath cycles.

2. 4-7-8 Breathing (Relaxing Breath):

- **How to Practice:**
    - Sit in a comfortable position.
    - Gently inhale through your nose until you reach the fourth mental count.
    - For seven counts, hold your breath.
    - Completely release the breath via your lips, counting to eight.
    - This cycle constitutes one breath. Repeat for several cycles.

3. Box Breathing (Square Breathing):

- **How to Practice:**
    - Take four deep breaths through your nose.
    - For four counts, hold your breath.
    - Take a full four breaths out through your mouth.
    - Take a moment to pause and hold your breath for four more counts.
    - Repeat the cycle for several rounds.

4. Alternate Nostril Breathing (Nadi Shodhana):

- **How to Practice:**
  - Sit comfortably with a straight spine.
  - Use your right thumb to close off your right nostril.
  - Inhale through your left nostril.
  - Close your left nostril with your right ring finger.
  - Release the right nostril and exhale.
  - Inhale through the right nostril.
  - Close the right nostril and exhale through the left.
  - This completes one cycle. Repeat for several cycles.

5. Resonant or Coherent Breathing:

- **How to Practice:**
  - Inhale and exhale slowly through your nose.
  - Aim for a comfortable and consistent breath rate, such as five to six breaths per minute.
  - Focus on making your inhales and exhales of equal duration.
  - Use a timer or paced breathing app for guidance.

6. Cleansing Breath (Three-Part Breath):

- **How to Practice:**
  - Sit comfortably with a straight spine.
  - Inhale deeply through your nose, filling your lower abdomen, then your chest, and finally your upper chest.
  - Exhale completely through your mouth, releasing air from the upper chest, chest, and lower abdomen.
  - Repeat for several breath cycles.

7. Sama Vritti (Equal Breathing):

- **How to Practice:**
  - Inhale through your nose for a count of four.
  - Exhale through your nose for a count of four.
  - Ensure that the inhale and exhale are of equal duration.

- Gradually increase the count as you become more comfortable.

TIPS FOR DEEP BREATHING:

- **Comfort:** Find a quiet and comfortable place to practice.
- **Posture:** Sit or lie down with a straight spine to allow for optimal breathing.
- **Focus:** Concentrate on the breath and try to let go of distracting thoughts.
- **Regular Practice:** Incorporate deep breathing into your daily routine for ongoing benefits.
- **Adapt to Your Needs:** Adjust the pace and duration to suit your comfort level.
- **Mindfulness:** Be present in the moment, paying attention to the sensations of breathing.

Deep breathing exercises are versatile and can be practiced almost anywhere. They are especially helpful during moments of stress, before bedtime, or as part of a mindfulness routine. Consistent practice can contribute to a greater sense of calm, reduced anxiety, and improved overall well-being.

CHAPTER FIVE
HOLISTIC APPROACHES TO DEPRESSION

Holistic approaches to depression involve addressing the condition on multiple levels—physical, mental, emotional, and spiritual. These approaches aim to promote overall well-being and address underlying factors contributing to depression. It's crucial to note that these methods can complement traditional treatments, and individuals should consult with healthcare professionals for comprehensive care. Here are holistic approaches that may be considered:

1. Nutrition and Diet:

- **Balanced Diet:** Focus on a well-balanced diet rich in whole foods, including fruits, vegetables, lean proteins, and whole grains.
- **Nutrient Supplementation:** Consider supplements like omega-3 fatty acids, vitamin D, and B-vitamins, which are linked to mood regulation.
- **Limit Sugar and Processed Foods:** Reduce intake of refined sugars and processed foods, as they can negatively impact mood.

2. Exercise and Movement:

- **Regular Physical Activity:** Engage in regular exercise, which has been shown to release endorphins, improve mood, and reduce symptoms of depression.
- **Mindful Movement Practices:** Include practices like yoga or tai chi that combine physical activity with mindfulness.

3. Mindfulness and Meditation:

- **Mindfulness Meditation:** Practice mindfulness meditation to develop awareness of thoughts and emotions, reducing stress and enhancing emotional well-being.
- **Mindful Breathing:** Incorporate deep breathing exercises and mindful breathing techniques to promote relaxation.

4. Holistic Psychotherapy:

- **Mind-Body Approaches:** Holistic psychotherapy may integrate traditional talk therapy with mind-body approaches such as mindfulness, meditation, and art therapy.
- **Exploration of Root Causes:** Addressing underlying emotional and psychological factors contributing to depression.

5. Herbal Remedies:

- **St. John's Wort:** This herb has been studied for its potential antidepressant effects, although its use should be approached with caution and under the guidance of a healthcare professional.
- **Lavender Oil:** Lavender aromatherapy or supplements may have calming effects.

6. Acupuncture:

- **Energy Balance:** Acupuncture, an ancient Chinese practice, is believed to balance the flow of energy (Qi) in the body. Some studies suggest it may be beneficial for depression.
- **Holistic Assessment:** Acupuncturists often consider lifestyle factors and emotional well-being in their treatments.

7. Yoga and Tai Chi:

- **Mind-Body Connection:** Practices like yoga and tai chi emphasize the mind-body connection, promoting relaxation, reducing stress, and improving mood.

- **Physical Activity:** Additionally, these practices involve physical activity, which can contribute to overall well-being.

8. Nature Therapy:

- **Outdoor Activities:** Spend time in nature, as exposure to natural environments has been linked to improved mood and mental health.
- **Ecotherapy:** Engage in activities that connect with the natural world, such as gardening or hiking.

9. Social Connection:

- **Support Systems:** Cultivate strong social connections and a support system. Share feelings and experiences with trusted friends or family.
- **Group Activities:** Join group activities, clubs, or support groups to foster a sense of community.

10. Sleep Hygiene:

- **Quality Sleep:** Prioritize healthy sleep habits, ensuring sufficient and restful sleep each night.
- **Sleep Routine:** Establish a regular sleep routine and create a comfortable sleep environment.

11. Cognitive Behavioral Therapy (CBT):

- **Cognitive Restructuring:** CBT focuses on identifying and challenging negative thought patterns, helping individuals develop more positive and adaptive thinking.
- **Behavioral Activation:** Encourages engagement in positive and fulfilling activities.

12. Spiritual Practices:

- **Mind-Body-Spirit Connection:** Engage in spiritual practices that resonate with personal beliefs, such as prayer, meditation, or connecting with a higher power.
- **Sense of Purpose:** Cultivate a sense of purpose and meaning in life.

13. Art and Music Therapy:

- **Creative Expression:** Art and music therapy can provide a creative outlet for expressing emotions and fostering self-discovery.
- **Emotional Release:** Engaging in creative activities may contribute to emotional release and stress reduction.

Holistic approaches to depression acknowledge the complexity of the condition and seek to address various aspects of an individual's life. It's essential for individuals experiencing depression to work collaboratively with healthcare professionals to create a comprehensive and personalized treatment plan. This plan may involve a combination of traditional medical treatments and holistic approaches to promote holistic well-being.

ACUPUNCTURE AND ITS EMOTIONAL BENEFITS

Acupuncture is a traditional Chinese medicine that includes inserting tiny needles into certain body sites. While it's commonly known for its physical benefits, such as pain relief and improved circulation, acupuncture is also believed to have emotional and mental health benefits. Here are some ways in which acupuncture may contribute to emotional well-being:

1. Stress Reduction:

- **Calming Effect:** Acupuncture is thought to stimulate the release of endorphins, the body's natural "feel-good" chemicals. This can lead to a sense of relaxation and calmness.

- **Regulation of the Nervous System:** Acupuncture may influence the autonomic nervous system, helping to balance the sympathetic (fight-or-flight) and parasympathetic (rest-and-digest) branches. This balance is crucial for stress management.

2. Anxiety and Depression:

- **Endorphin Release:** The release of endorphins during acupuncture may not only reduce physical pain but also contribute to a more positive mood.
- **Regulation of Neurotransmitters:** Some studies suggest that acupuncture may influence the levels of neurotransmitters such as serotonin and dopamine, which play key roles in mood regulation.

3. Improved Sleep:

- **Relaxation Response:** Acupuncture may help induce a relaxation response, promoting better sleep quality.
- **Regulation of Circadian Rhythms:** By influencing the nervous system, acupuncture could contribute to the regulation of circadian rhythms, positively impacting sleep patterns.

4. Balancing Emotional Energy:

- **Traditional Chinese Medicine (TCM) Perspective:** In TCM, emotions are seen as interconnected with the body's energy (Qi) flow. Acupuncture aims to balance this energy, addressing emotional imbalances.
- **Meridian Stimulation:** Acupuncture points are located along meridians, and stimulation of specific points is believed to affect the flow of energy, promoting emotional well-being.

5. Reduction of Cortisol Levels:

- **Stress Hormone Regulation:** Acupuncture may play a role in regulating cortisol, the body's primary stress hormone. Elevated cortisol levels are associated with chronic stress and can negatively impact mental health.

6. Enhanced Mind-Body Connection:

- **Focused Awareness:** The practice of acupuncture often involves intentional focus on the body and breath, fostering a mind-body connection.
- **Body Awareness:** By increasing awareness of bodily sensations, acupuncture may help individuals become more attuned to their emotions and stressors.

7. Support for Emotional Healing:

- **Holistic Approach:** Acupuncture is often considered a holistic approach to health, addressing both physical and emotional aspects.
- **Facilitation of Self-Healing:** Traditional Chinese Medicine views acupuncture as a way to support the body's natural healing processes, which can extend to emotional healing.

8. Mood Regulation:

- **Balancing Yin and Yang:** In TCM philosophy, acupuncture aims to balance the opposing forces of yin and yang, contributing to overall harmony and balance, including emotional balance.
- **Individualized Approach:** Acupuncture treatments are often personalized based on an individual's unique health and emotional needs.

9. Coping with Trauma:

- **Trauma-Informed Acupuncture:** Some practitioners offer trauma-informed acupuncture, recognizing the potential role it can play in supporting individuals dealing with trauma.
- **Safe and Non-Verbal:** Acupuncture provides a non-verbal form of therapy, which can be beneficial for individuals who may find it challenging to express their emotions verbally.

10. Mindfulness and Present-Moment Awareness:

- **Intentional Focus:** The process of acupuncture often involves intentional focus and presence, fostering mindfulness.
- **Stress Reduction through Mindfulness:** Mindfulness practices are known to reduce stress, and acupuncture provides an avenue for cultivating mindfulness.

While many people report emotional benefits from acupuncture, individual responses can vary. It's important to approach acupuncture as a complementary therapy and consult with a qualified healthcare professional, such as a licensed acupuncturist, especially when integrating it into a broader mental health treatment plan. Acupuncture should be seen as part of a holistic approach to emotional well-being, which may also include lifestyle changes, psychotherapy, and other supportive interventions.

MASSAGE THERAPY FOR STRESS REDUCTION

Massage therapy is a popular and effective approach for stress reduction and relaxation. The physical manipulation of muscles and soft tissues not only feels good but also has several physiological and psychological benefits. Here's how massage therapy can help with stress reduction:

1. Muscle Relaxation:

- **Tension Release:** Massage helps release muscle tension and tightness, which often accumulates due to stress.
- **Improved Flexibility:** By relaxing muscles, massage can enhance flexibility and joint mobility.

2. Stress Hormone Regulation:

- **Cortisol Reduction:** Massage has been shown to reduce cortisol, the stress hormone, leading to a sense of relaxation.

- **Endorphin Release:** Massage stimulates the release of endorphins, the body's natural mood enhancers, promoting a sense of well-being.

3. Improved Blood Circulation:

- **Enhanced Oxygen and Nutrient Delivery:** Massage increases blood flow, ensuring that muscles receive more oxygen and nutrients, promoting overall health.
- **Toxin Removal:** Improved circulation aids in the removal of waste products and toxins from the body.

4. Lowering Blood Pressure:

- **Relaxation Response:** Massage induces the relaxation response, which can help lower blood pressure.
- **Reduced Sympathetic Nervous System Activity:** Massage may decrease activity in the sympathetic nervous system associated with the "fight or flight" response.

5. Improved Sleep Quality:

- **Melatonin Release:** Massage has been linked to an increase in serotonin and melatonin levels, hormones associated with sleep regulation.
- **Relaxing Effect:** The calming effect of massage can contribute to improved sleep quality.

6. Stress-Related Pain Relief:

- **Headache and Migraine Relief:** Massage can help alleviate tension headaches and migraines often associated with stress.
- **Reduced Muscular Pain:** Chronic stress can contribute to muscle pain, and massage provides relief by relaxing tight muscles.

7. Enhanced Mood:

- **Serotonin and Dopamine Release:** Massage stimulates the release of serotonin and dopamine, neurotransmitters that contribute to feelings of happiness and well-being.
- **Reduced Anxiety and Depression Symptoms:** Regular massage sessions have been associated with reductions in symptoms of anxiety and depression.

8. Mind-Body Connection:

- **Mindful Awareness:** Massage encourages individuals to be present and aware of their bodies, fostering a mind-body connection.
- **Reduced Mental Stress:** The focus on the physical sensations during a massage session can distract from mental stressors.

9. Immune System Support:

- **Increased White Blood Cell Activity:** Some studies suggest that massage can enhance the activity of white blood cells, supporting the immune system.
- **Reduced Inflammatory Markers:** Massage has been associated with decreased levels of inflammatory markers in the body.

10. Promotion of Relaxation Response:

- **Activation of Parasympathetic Nervous System:** Massage stimulates the parasympathetic nervous system, promoting the body's "rest and digest" response.
- **Balancing Stress Response:** Regular massage may help balance the overall stress response in the body.

TIPS FOR MAXIMIZING THE BENEFITS OF MASSAGE THERAPY:

- **Regular Sessions:** Consistency is key. Regular massage sessions, whether weekly or monthly, can maximize the cumulative benefits.

- **Open Communication:** Communicate openly with your massage therapist about your stress levels, areas of tension, and preferences for pressure.
- **Hydration:** Drink plenty of water after a massage to help flush out toxins released during the session.
- **Post-Massage Relaxation:** Allow time for relaxation after a massage to fully enjoy the calming effects.
- **Self-Care Practices:** Complement massage therapy with other self-care practices, such as deep breathing, meditation, or gentle exercise.

It's important to note that while massage therapy can be a valuable component of stress management, individuals with certain health conditions or concerns should consult with healthcare professionals before starting a massage therapy regimen. Additionally, choosing a licensed and experienced massage therapist ensures a safe and effective experience.

AROMATHERAPY FOR MOOD ENHANCEMENT

Aromatherapy is a holistic healing practice that uses the natural scents of essential oils to promote overall well-being, including mood enhancement. Essential oils, derived from various plant parts, contain aromatic compounds that can influence the mind and body when inhaled or applied to the skin. Here are some popular essential oils and ways in which aromatherapy can be used for mood enhancement:

1. Lavender:

- **Mood Benefits:** Lavender is known for its calming and soothing properties, making it useful for reducing stress and promoting relaxation.
- **How to Use:** Diffuse lavender oil in a room, add a few drops to a bath, or use it in a personal inhaler.

2. Citrus Oils (Orange, Lemon, Grapefruit):

- **Mood Benefits:** Citrus oils are often uplifting and refreshing, helping to boost mood and energy levels.
- **How to Use:** Diffuse citrus oils, add a few drops to a diffuser necklace, or inhale directly from the bottle.

3. Peppermint:

- **Mood Benefits:** Peppermint is invigorating and can help improve focus and mental clarity.
- **How to Use:** Diffuse peppermint oil, inhale directly, or add a few drops to a tissue and place it near your workspace.

4. Chamomile:

- **Mood Benefits:** Chamomile is known for its calming and relaxing effects, promoting a sense of tranquility.
- **How to Use:** Diffuse chamomile oil, add a few drops to a warm bath, or use it in massage oil.

5. Ylang-Ylang:

- **Mood Benefits:** Ylang-ylang is often used for its mood-balancing properties, promoting feelings of joy and relaxation.
- **How to Use:** Diffuse ylang-ylang oil, add a few drops to a carrier oil for massage, or use it in a personal inhaler.

6. Rosemary:

- **Mood Benefits:** Rosemary is invigorating and can help improve mental clarity and concentration.
- **How to Use:** Diffuse rosemary oil, inhale directly, or add a few drops to a warm bath.

7. Bergamot:

- **Mood Benefits:** Bergamot is known for its uplifting and calming effects, making it useful for stress reduction.
- **How to Use:** Diffuse bergamot oil, add a few drops to a diffuser bracelet, or use it in a room spray.

8. Frankincense:

- **Mood Benefits:** Frankincense is often used for its grounding and centering properties, promoting a sense of peace.
- **How to Use:** Diffuse frankincense oil, apply a diluted solution to pulse points, or add a few drops to a meditation practice.

9. Cedarwood:

- **Mood Benefits:** Cedarwood is grounding and can help create a sense of stability and calm.
- **How to Use:** Diffuse cedarwood oil, add a few drops to a diffuser necklace, or use it in a homemade room spray.

10. Eucalyptus:

- **Mood Benefits:** Eucalyptus is invigorating and can help clear the mind, especially during times of congestion or fatigue.
- **How to Use:** Diffuse eucalyptus oil, inhale directly, or add a few drops to a bowl of hot water for steam inhalation.

TIPS FOR AROMATHERAPY FOR MOOD ENHANCEMENT:

- **Use a Diffuser:** A diffuser disperses essential oils into the air, providing a continuous and gentle release of aromas.
- **Inhalation:** Inhale essential oils directly from the bottle, use a personal inhaler, or add a few drops to a tissue.
- **Topical Application:** Dilute essential oils in carrier oil and apply to pulse points, such as wrists and temples.

- **Baths:** Add a few drops of essential oil to a warm bath for a relaxing and mood-enhancing experience.
- **Massage:** Combine essential oils with carrier oil for a soothing and mood-balancing massage.
- **Create Blends:** Experiment with creating your own essential oil blends to find combinations that resonate with your mood preferences.

It's important to note that individual responses to aromatherapy can vary, and some people may be sensitive to certain essential oils. Always follow safety guidelines, use high-quality oils, and consider personal preferences when exploring aromatherapy for mood enhancement. If you have any existing health conditions or concerns, consult with a healthcare professional before incorporating aromatherapy into your routine.

CHAPTER SIX
SOCIAL SUPPORT AND CONNECTIONS

Social support and connections play a crucial role in mental health and overall well-being. Human beings are inherently social creatures, and positive social interactions contribute significantly to emotional resilience and a sense of belonging. Here are seven key aspects of social support and connections that impact mental health:

1. Emotional Support:

- **Listening and Understanding:** Having someone who listens and understands your emotions can provide comfort and validation.
- **Expressing Feelings:** Sharing feelings with a supportive friend or family member can alleviate emotional burdens.

2. Practical Support:

- **Tangible Assistance:** Practical support involves concrete help with tasks, such as running errands, cooking meals, or assisting with daily responsibilities.
- **Shared Responsibilities:** Collaborating on responsibilities can reduce stress and create a sense of shared effort.

3. Companionship:

- **Shared Activities:** Engaging in activities with friends or loved ones fosters a sense of companionship and connection.
- **Quality Time:** Spending quality time together strengthens bonds and provides opportunities for joy and shared experiences.

4. Sense of Belonging:

- **Inclusion and Acceptance:** Feeling accepted and included in social circles promotes a sense of belonging.
- **Community Connection:** Being part of a community or social group provides a broader sense of identity and support.

5. Reducing Isolation:

- **Social Interaction:** Regular social contact helps combat feelings of isolation and loneliness.
- **Virtual Connections:** In the digital age, online connections can also play a role in reducing isolation.

6. Conflict Resolution:

- **Open Communication:** Healthy relationships involve open communication to address conflicts and misunderstandings.
- **Conflict Resolution Skills:** Learning effective conflict resolution skills enhances the quality of social connections.

7. Building Resilience:

- **Coping Together:** Having a support system helps individuals cope with life's challenges and setbacks.
- **Sharing Perspectives:** Different perspectives within a social network contribute to a more resilient mindset.

TIPS FOR CULTIVATING SOCIAL SUPPORT:

1. **Nurture Relationships:** Invest time and effort into building and maintaining positive relationships.
2. **Communicate Effectively:** Be open and honest in your communication, expressing your needs and feelings.
3. **Active Listening:** Practice active listening to understand others and make them feel heard.

4. **Be Reliable:** Being reliable and trustworthy strengthens the foundation of relationships.
5. **Seek Support:** Don't hesitate to reach out when you need support or someone to talk to.
6. **Participate in Social Activities:** Engage in social activities, whether in person or virtually, to foster connections.
7. **Join Communities:** Participate in clubs, groups, or organizations aligned with your interests for shared experiences.
8. **Show Empathy:** Demonstrate empathy and understanding toward others, creating a supportive environment.
9. **Set Boundaries:** Establish healthy boundaries in relationships to ensure mutual respect and well-being.
10. **Celebrate Achievements:** Acknowledge and celebrate both your own and others' achievements.

IMPACT ON MENTAL HEALTH:

1. **Stress Reduction:** Social support helps buffer the impact of stress, providing coping mechanisms.
2. **Improved Mood:** Positive social interactions contribute to a positive mood and emotional well-being.
3. **Increased Resilience:** Social connections enhance resilience, helping individuals bounce back from challenges.
4. **Lower Risk of Mental Health Issues:** Strong social support is associated with a lower risk of mental health issues.
5. **Enhanced Self-Esteem:** Feeling valued and supported boosts self-esteem and self-worth.

WARNING SIGNS OF INSUFFICIENT SOCIAL SUPPORT:

1. **Isolation:** Persistent social withdrawal or isolation.
2. **Feelings of Loneliness:** Chronic feelings of loneliness and disconnection.
3. **Increased Stress:** Overwhelming stress without a supportive outlet.
4. **Emotional Distress:** Frequent emotional distress without available support.

5. **Depression and Anxiety:** Symptoms of depression or anxiety without adequate support.

In conclusion, fostering social support and connections is a vital aspect of mental health. Building and maintaining positive relationships contribute to emotional well-being, stress reduction, and overall life satisfaction. Prioritizing social connections and seeking support when needed are essential steps toward creating a supportive and resilient network. If individuals find it challenging to establish or maintain social connections, reaching out to mental health professionals or support groups can be beneficial.

BUILDING A SUPPORT SYSTEM

Building a strong support system is a crucial aspect of maintaining mental health and well-being. A support system consists of individuals who offer emotional support, practical assistance, and positive connections. Here are steps to help you build and strengthen your support system:

1. Identify Potential Supporters:

- **Family and Friends:** Consider close family members and friends who have demonstrated support in the past.
- **Colleagues:** Build supportive relationships at work with colleagues who understand your challenges.
- **Community and Social Groups:** Join clubs, organizations, or social groups that align with your interests to meet like-minded individuals.

2. Cultivate Healthy Relationships:

- **Positive Interactions:** Prioritize relationships with individuals who contribute positively to your life.
- **Reciprocity:** Seek relationships where there is a mutual exchange of support and care.

3. Communicate Your Needs:

- **Open Communication:** Clearly communicate your needs, feelings, and expectations to potential supporters.
- **Express Vulnerability:** Allow yourself to be vulnerable when sharing your thoughts and emotions.

4. Be a Supportive Friend:

- **Reciprocal Support:** Offer support to others in your network, fostering a culture of mutual assistance.
- **Active Listening:** Practice active listening to understand the needs and concerns of those around you.

5. Diversify Your Support System:

- **Different Types of Support:** Seek support from various sources, including emotional, practical, and informational.
- **Professional Support:** Consider incorporating mental health professionals into your support system if needed.

6. Join Supportive Communities:

- **Online Groups:** Explore online communities and forums where individuals share similar experiences or challenges.
- **Local Meetups:** Attend local meetups or support groups for face-to-face connections.

7. Participate in Social Activities:

- **Shared Interests:** Engage in activities that align with your interests to meet like-minded individuals.
- **Classes and Workshops:** Take classes or attend workshops to connect with people who share common goals.

8. Nurture Existing Relationships:

- **Quality Time:** Spend quality time with friends and family to strengthen existing bonds.
- **Celebrate Milestones:** Acknowledge and celebrate important milestones and achievements together.

9. Set Boundaries:

- **Healthy Boundaries:** Establish clear and healthy boundaries to ensure balanced and respectful relationships.
- **Respect Personal Space:** Recognize and respect the need for personal space and autonomy.

10. Practice Self-Disclosure:

- **Share Your Story:** When appropriate, share your experiences and challenges to deepen connections.
- **Encourage Openness:** Encourage others in your support system to share their experiences as well.

11. Utilize Technology:

- **Stay Connected:** Use technology to stay connected with friends and family, especially if they are geographically distant.
- **Virtual Support:** Leverage video calls, messaging apps, and social media for ongoing communication.

12. Seek Professional Guidance:

- **Therapy or Counseling:** Consider seeking therapy or counseling to explore challenges and receive professional support.
- **Support Groups:** Join support groups led by mental health professionals for a structured and supportive environment.

13. Evaluate and Adjust:

- **Assess Relationships:** Regularly assess the quality and effectiveness of your support system.
- **Make Adjustments:** If needed, make adjustments by adding new connections or reassessing existing ones.

14. Be Patient:

- **Building Takes Time:** Building a strong support system is a gradual process that takes time and effort.
- **Cultivate Patience:** Be patient with yourself and the process of establishing meaningful connections.

15. Consider Professional Assistance:

- **Therapy or Counseling:** If building a support system feels challenging, consider seeking the guidance of a therapist or counselor.
- **Life Coaching:** Explore life coaching for assistance in setting and achieving personal and relationship goals.

Building a support system is an ongoing process that involves both nurturing existing connections and being open to new ones. Remember that the quality of your support system is more important than the quantity. A small group of supportive and trustworthy individuals can have a significant positive impact on your mental health. Don't hesitate to reach out for professional guidance if you encounter challenges in building or maintaining your support system.

THE IMPACT OF POSITIVE RELATIONSHIPS

Positive relationships have a profound impact on mental and emotional well-being, contributing significantly to an individual's overall quality of life. These relationships, characterized by mutual support, trust, and shared positive experiences, play a crucial role in fostering happiness, resilience, and a sense of belonging. Here are some key ways in which positive relationships can positively impact individuals:

1. Emotional Well-Being:

- **Support and Validation:** Positive relationships provide emotional support, offering a safe space for expressing feelings and concerns.
- **Validation and Understanding:** Feeling understood and validated by others contributes to emotional well-being.

2. Reduced Stress Levels:

- **Buffering Stress:** Supportive relationships act as a buffer against stress, helping individuals cope with life's challenges.
- **Cortisol Regulation:** Positive interactions in relationships can regulate cortisol levels, reducing the physiological impact of stress.

3. Increased Resilience:

- **Mutual Support:** Positive relationships provide a foundation of mutual support, enhancing an individual's ability to bounce back from setbacks.
- **Shared Coping Mechanisms:** Coping with difficulties together strengthens resilience.

4. Enhanced Self-Esteem:

- **Affirmation and Encouragement:** Positive relationships contribute to feelings of affirmation and encouragement, boosting self-esteem.
- **Celebration of Achievements:** Celebrating personal and shared achievements reinforces a positive self-image.

5. Improved Mental Health:

- **Emotional Regulation:** Supportive relationships contribute to emotional regulation and stability.
- **Reduced Risk of Mental Health Issues:** Positive social connections are associated with a lower risk of mental health issues, such as depression and anxiety.

6. Greater Life Satisfaction:

- **Shared Experiences:** Positive relationships provide opportunities for shared experiences, contributing to overall life satisfaction.
- **Sense of Purpose:** Feeling connected to others gives life a sense of purpose and meaning.

7. Physical Health Benefits:

- **Immune System Support:** Positive relationships are linked to a stronger immune system and overall better physical health.
- **Longevity:** Strong social connections are associated with increased longevity.

8. Improved Coping Mechanisms:

- **Shared Problem-Solving:** Positive relationships offer collaborative problem-solving, making it easier to navigate challenges.
- **Diverse Perspectives:** Different perspectives within a social network contribute to more creative and effective problem-solving.

9. Sense of Belonging:

- **Inclusion and Acceptance:** Positive relationships foster a sense of belonging and acceptance.
- **Community Connection:** Feeling connected to a community or group provides a broader sense of identity.

10. Increased Empathy and Compassion:

- **Reciprocal Care:** Positive relationships cultivate empathy and compassion, leading to a more caring and supportive community.
- **Understanding Others:** Understanding and supporting others in relationships foster a sense of interconnectedness.

11. Better Communication Skills:

- **Open Communication:** Positive relationships often involve effective communication, enhancing the quality of interactions.
- **Conflict Resolution:** Navigating conflicts within positive relationships contributes to the development of strong communication and conflict resolution skills.

12. Positive Influence on Behavior:

- **Healthier Lifestyle Choices:** Positive relationships can influence individuals to make healthier lifestyle choices.
- **Encouragement for Positive Habits:** Encouragement and shared goals within relationships contribute to positive habits.

13. Supportive Networks During Challenges:

- **Shared Burdens:** Positive relationships provide a network of support during challenging times.
- **Collective Strength:** Facing challenges together with the support of others increases collective strength.

14. Increased Motivation:

- **Shared Goals:** Positive relationships often involve shared goals and aspirations, providing motivation.
- **Encouragement:** Encouragement from others in achieving personal and professional goals boosts motivation.

15. Happiness and Joy:

- **Shared Joy:** Positive relationships contribute to shared moments of happiness and joy.
- **Emotional Fulfillment:** Positive connections bring emotional fulfillment and a sense of joy in day-to-day life.

CULTIVATING POSITIVE RELATIONSHIPS:

1. **Prioritize Quality Over Quantity:** Focus on the depth and quality of relationships rather than the number of connections.
2. **Open Communication:** Foster open and honest communication to build trust and understanding.
3. **Mutual Respect:** Cultivate relationships based on mutual respect and appreciation.
4. **Reciprocity:** Encourage a give-and-take dynamic, where support and care are mutual.
5. **Set Healthy Boundaries:** Establish and respect healthy boundaries within relationships.
6. **Express Gratitude:** Regularly express gratitude for the positive relationships in your life.
7. **Be Present:** Practice being present and fully engaged in your interactions.
8. **Apologize and Forgive:** Apologize when necessary, and practice forgiveness to maintain healthy relationships.
9. **Invest Time and Effort:** Building and maintaining positive relationships requires time and effort.
10. **Seek Professional Support:** If needed, seek the guidance of mental health professionals for relationship support.

Positive relationships contribute significantly to an individual's mental health and overall well-being. Investing time and energy in nurturing these connections is a valuable aspect of a fulfilling and satisfying life. If individuals find it challenging to build positive relationships or navigate interpersonal challenges, seeking the guidance of a mental health professional can provide valuable insights and support.

JOINING SUPPORTIVE COMMUNITIES

Joining supportive communities can have numerous positive effects on your well-being, providing a sense of connection, understanding, and shared experiences. Here are practical steps to guide you in joining and engaging with supportive communities:

1. Identify Your Interests and Needs:

- Define your interests, challenges, or goals.
- Consider what type of community would best address your needs.

2. Explore In-Person and Online Options:

- Look for local meetups, clubs, or organizations related to your interests.
- Explore online forums, social media groups, or virtual communities.

3. Research Communities:

- Review community values, guidelines, and mission statements.
- Check for user reviews or testimonials to gauge the community's atmosphere.

4. Join Relevant Social Media Groups:

- Join Facebook groups, Reddit communities, or other platforms aligned with your interests.
- Engage in discussions and contribute positively to build connections.

5. Attend Local Events or Meetups:

- Check local event platforms for gatherings related to your interests.
- Attend events to meet people in person and deepen connections.

6. Contribute Positively:

- Share your experiences, insights, or resources in discussions.
- Offer support and encouragement to others in the community.

7. Create Your Own Community:

- Initiate gatherings or online groups if you can't find a community that fits.
- Moderate effectively to maintain a positive environment.

8. Attend Workshops or Classes:

- Join communities centered around learning new skills or attending workshops.
- Engage in shared learning experiences to connect with like-minded individuals.

9. Be Open to Diverse Perspectives:

- Embrace diversity within the community.
- Practice respect and empathy for different backgrounds and viewpoints.

10. Practice Consistency:

- Regularly participate in community activities, discussions, or events.
- Schedule check-ins to strengthen the sense of community.

11. Set Healthy Boundaries:

- Respect others' boundaries and communicate your own.
- Foster a safe and respectful environment for interactions.

12. Seek Professional Support If Needed:

- Consider therapeutic communities or support groups led by mental health professionals.
- Combine community support with professional guidance for a holistic approach.

13. Share and Celebrate Achievements:

- Share your achievements and milestones within the community.
- Celebrate the successes of others to foster a positive atmosphere.

14. Maintain Flexibility:

- Adapt to changes within the community.
- Explore new communities if your interests evolve.

15. Enjoy the Journey:

- Cultivate enjoyment in the process of building connections.
- Value the relationships formed and the support received from the community.

16. Participate Actively:

- Engage in discussions, activities, or projects within the community.
- Active participation strengthens your connection with the community.

17. Be Supportive and Empathetic:

- Offer support to others facing challenges.
- Practice empathy to create a compassionate community environment.

18. Respect Privacy and Confidentiality:

- Respect the privacy and confidentiality of community members.
- Create a trustworthy environment for open sharing.

19. Celebrate Diversity:

- Appreciate the diversity of experiences, backgrounds, and perspectives.
- Create an inclusive community that welcomes people from various walks of life.

20. Seek Growth and Learning:

- View community involvement as an opportunity for personal growth.
- Be open to learning from others and expanding your understanding.

Remember that the process of building connections and finding the right community may take time. Be patient, and allow relationships to develop organically. Enjoy the journey of discovering new connections, gaining support, and contributing positively to the communities you join.

CHAPTER SEVEN
LIMITING NEGATIVE INFLUENCES

Limiting negative influences is an essential aspect of maintaining positive mental health and well-being. Negative influences can come in various forms, including toxic relationships, exposure to negative media, or engaging in self-destructive behaviors. Here are practical steps to help you limit negative influences and foster a more positive environment:

1. Identify Negative Influences:

- Reflect on your daily life and relationships to identify sources of negativity.
- Recognize patterns of negative thinking, behaviors, or relationships.

2. Evaluate Relationships:

- Evaluate how your connections affect your overall health.
- Identify relationships that consistently bring negativity or stress into your life.

3. Establish Boundaries:

- Set clear and healthy boundaries with individuals who contribute negatively to your life.
- Communicate your boundaries assertively and stick to them.

4. Limit Exposure to Negative Media:

- Be mindful of the media you consume, including news, social media, and entertainment.
- Limit exposure to content that induces stress, anxiety, or negative emotions.

5. Cultivate Positive Connections:

- Give connections that encourage and support you top priority.
- Foster connections with individuals who share positive values and perspectives.

6. Practice Self-Reflection:

- Regularly reflect on your own thoughts, beliefs, and behaviors.
- Recognize and confront limiting beliefs or negative self-talk.

7. Engage in Positive Activities:

- Fill your time with activities that bring joy, fulfillment, and positivity.
- Pursue hobbies, engage in creative outlets, or participate in activities that promote well-being.

8. Seek Professional Support:

- If negative influences stem from deep-rooted issues, consider seeking therapy or counseling.
- A mental health professional can provide guidance in addressing underlying issues.

9. Create a Supportive Environment:

- Surround yourself with a positive and supportive environment at home and work.
- Decorate your space with items that bring joy, and make your surroundings conducive to well-being.

10. Learn to Say No:

- Practice saying no to commitments or activities that drain your energy.
- Prioritize your well-being by not overextending yourself.

11. Mindful Social Media Use:

- Be deliberate in how you utilize social media.
- Unfollow or mute accounts that contribute to negativity and comparison.

12. Evaluate Personal Habits:

- Assess your daily habits, including sleep, nutrition, and exercise.
- Ensure that your habits contribute to positive physical and mental health.

13. Practice Gratitude:

- Make it a habit to be grateful by concentrating on the good things in your life.
- Regularly express appreciation for the people and experiences that bring joy.

14. Build a Positive Routine:

- Establish a daily routine that includes activities promoting well-being.
- Consistency in positive habits can help counteract negative influences.

15. Challenge Negative Thoughts:

- Actively challenge negative thoughts and cognitive distortions.
- Swap out pessimistic ideas for more sensible and optimistic ones.

16. Monitor Self-Talk:

- Pay attention to your internal dialogue.
- Replace self-critical or negative self-talk with affirming and compassionate language.

17. Engage in Stress-Reducing Practices:

- Incorporate stress-reducing practices into your routine, such as mindfulness, meditation, or deep breathing exercises.
- These practices can help manage and mitigate the impact of negative influences.

18. Educate Yourself:

- Stay informed about the impact of negativity on mental health.
- Educate yourself on healthy coping mechanisms and strategies.

19. Connect with Positive Communities:

- Join communities or groups that share positive values and interests.
- Surrounding yourself with positivity can create a supportive social network.

20. Celebrate Progress:

- Acknowledge and celebrate your efforts in limiting negative influences.
- Recognize the progress you make in creating a more positive and uplifting life.

Limiting negative influences is an ongoing process that requires self-awareness and intentional choices. By taking proactive steps to create a positive environment, you can contribute to your mental well-being and build a foundation for a more fulfilling life. If you find it challenging to manage negative influences on your own, seeking guidance from a mental health professional can provide additional support and strategies tailored to your individual needs.

MANAGING SOCIAL MEDIA AND SCREEN TIME

Managing social media and screen time is crucial for maintaining a healthy balance in your life and protecting your mental well-being. Excessive use of digital devices, social media, and online platforms can contribute to stress, anxiety, and a range of negative effects. Here are practical tips for managing social media and screen time:

1. Set Boundaries:

- Establish clear boundaries for your screen time, both on social media and other digital activities.
- Define specific time limits for daily usage.

2. Schedule Screen-Free Time:

- Set out particular periods of the day for activities that don't involve screens.
- Use this time for hobbies, outdoor activities, or connecting with loved ones.

3. Create a Technology-Free Zone:

- Designate certain areas in your home, such as the bedroom or dining area, as technology-free zones.
- This helps create spaces for relaxation and face-to-face interactions.

4. Turn Off Notifications:

- Turn off unused notifications on your electronics to cut down on interruptions.
- Check messages and updates at specific times rather than reacting to constant alerts.

5. Establish a Social Media Schedule:

- Set specific times during the day to check and engage with social media.
- Avoid mindless scrolling by being intentional about your usage.

6. Use Apps to Limit Screen Time:

- Explore apps that help you monitor and limit your screen time.
- Set daily or weekly usage goals to stay accountable.

7. Prioritize Real-Life Connections:

- Devote time to establishing and maintaining relationships in real life.
- Plan in-person meetups or phone calls to maintain meaningful connections.

8. Practice Mindful Consumption:

- Pay attention to the stuff you click on and read on social media.
- Unfollow accounts that promote comparison or criticism.

9. Curate Your Social Media Feed:

- Adopt accounts that uplift, inform, or make you smile.
- Regularly review and curate your social media feed to align with positive content.

10. Set Screen Time Limits for Children:

- Establish age-appropriate screen time limits for children.
- Encourage a balance between screen activities and outdoor play.

11. Use the 20-20-20 Rule:

• To lessen eye strain, observe the 20-20-20 rule, which states that you should gaze at anything 20 feet away for at least 20 seconds every 20 minutes.

12. Create a Tech-Free Wind Down Routine:

- Establish a tech-free wind-down routine before bedtime.

- Avoid screens at least an hour before sleeping to promote better sleep quality.

13. Practice Digital Detox Days:

- Dedicate occasional days or weekends to a digital detox.
- Take a break from screens and do things offline.

14. Set App Time Limits:

- Many devices allow you to set app-specific time limits.
- Utilize these features to control your usage of particular apps.

15. Educate Yourself on Digital Well-Being:

- Stay informed about the impact of excessive screen time on mental health.
- Educate yourself on digital well-being practices and incorporate them into your routine.

16. Find Offline Hobbies:

- Cultivate offline hobbies and activities that don't involve screens.
- Engage in creative pursuits, exercise, or reading.

17. Be Intentional with Social Media Use:

- Use social media intentionally for positive interactions, learning, and connection.
- Avoid mindless scrolling by having a purpose for your online engagement.

18. Encourage Face-to-Face Interactions:

- Prioritize face-to-face interactions whenever possible.
- Use technology as a supplement to, not a replacement for, real-life connections.

19. Monitor Your Emotional Well-Being:

- Pay attention to how your screen time affects your mood and mental well-being.
- If you notice negative effects, consider adjustments to your digital habits.

20. Seek Professional Help if Needed:

- If you struggle to control your screen time and it negatively impacts your life, consider seeking guidance from a mental health professional.
- They are able to give you methods and assistance that are specific to your needs.

Managing social media and screen time is a personal journey, and finding the right balance requires self-awareness and intentional choices. By implementing these strategies, you can create a healthier relationship with technology and foster a more balanced and fulfilling lifestyle.

RECOGNIZING AND AVOIDING TOXIC RELATIONSHIPS

Recognizing and avoiding toxic relationships is crucial for maintaining your mental and emotional well-being. Toxic relationships can have detrimental effects on various aspects of your life, including self-esteem, mental health, and overall happiness. Here are key signs to help you recognize toxic relationships and practical steps to avoid or navigate them:

SIGNS OF A TOXIC RELATIONSHIP:

1. **Lack of Respect:**
    - Disrespectful behavior, including verbal, emotional, or physical abuse.

- Ignoring boundaries and consistently violating your personal space.

2. **Constant Criticism:**
   - Continuous criticism, blame, or demeaning remarks.
   - Feeling like you are never good enough or constantly walking on eggshells.

3. **Manipulation and Control:**
   - Attempts to control or manipulate your thoughts, actions, or decisions.
   - Using guilt, threats, or coercion to get what they want.

4. **Lack of Support:**
   - Absence of emotional support during challenging times.
   - Disinterest in your goals, dreams, or well-being.

5. **Draining Energy:**
   - Feeling emotionally drained or exhausted after interacting with the person.
   - Constant negativity and pessimism.

6. **One-Sided Relationships:**
   - An unequal distribution of giving and receiving in the partnership.
   - Feeling like you are the only one making an effort to maintain the relationship.

7. **Consistent Drama:**
   - Regular conflicts and drama without resolution.
   - Creating unnecessary stress and chaos.

8. **Isolation:**
   - Attempts to isolate you from friends, family, or other support systems.
   - Controlling who you can and cannot spend time with.

9. **Gaslighting:**
   - Manipulating facts or denying events to make you doubt your perception or memory.
   - Holding you accountable for their acts or blaming you for their behavior.

10. **Jealousy and Envy:**
    - Constant jealousy or attempts to undermine your achievements.

- Competing instead of celebrating your successes.

PRACTICAL STEPS TO AVOID OR NAVIGATE TOXIC RELATIONSHIPS:

1. **Trust Your Instincts:**
   - Be mindful of your instincts regarding the partnership.
   - Trust your instinct if something feels off or unhealthy.
2. **Set Boundaries:**
   - Clearly define and communicate your boundaries.
   - Be firm in enforcing boundaries and don't tolerate violations.
3. **Communicate Openly:**
   - Express your feelings and concerns openly and honestly.
   - Encourage open communication in the relationship.
4. **Seek Support:**
   - Seek help from loved ones, friends, or a therapist.
   - Talk to a trusted person about your thoughts and experiences.
5. **Limit Contact:**
   - Reduce or limit contact with the person if possible.
   - Create distance to protect your well-being.
6. **Prioritize Self-Care:**
   - Focus on self-care activities that promote your mental and emotional health.
   - Put your health above continuing in a harmful relationship.
7. **Establish Consequences:**
   - Clearly communicate consequences for continued toxic behavior.
   - Be prepared to enforce consequences if necessary.
8. **Practice Assertiveness:**
   - Develop assertiveness skills to express your needs and stand up for yourself.
   - Avoid passive or aggressive communication styles.
9. **Educate Yourself:**
   - Learn about healthy relationships and red flags of toxicity.
   - Understanding the dynamics can empower you to make informed decisions.

10. **Create a Support Network:**

    • Create a network of allies and friends who are there for you.

    • Surround yourself with positive, uplifting people.
11. **Reflect on Patterns:**
    - Reflect on patterns in your relationships and identify recurring toxic behaviors.
    - Consider seeking therapy to explore and address underlying patterns.
12. **End the Relationship:**
    - If the toxicity persists and efforts to improve the relationship are unsuccessful, consider ending the relationship.
    - Prioritize your well-being and make decisions that support your mental health.
13. **Focus on Personal Growth:**
    - Devote time to your own development and betterment.
    - Build resilience and a strong sense of self-worth.
14. **Learn from Experiences:**
    - Use experiences from toxic relationships as learning opportunities.
    - Identify red flags early in future relationships.
15. **Legal and Safety Considerations:**
    - If the relationship involves physical abuse or poses a threat to your safety, seek legal help and involve law enforcement if necessary.
    - Put your safety and the safety of any relatives first.

Recognizing and avoiding toxic relationships is a crucial aspect of maintaining a healthy and fulfilling life. It may require courage and self-reflection, but prioritizing your well-being is essential. If you find it challenging to navigate toxic relationships on your own, consider seeking the support of a therapist or counselor who can provide guidance tailored to your specific situation.

SETTING BOUNDARIES FOR MENTAL HEALTH

A vital component of preserving one's general well-being and mental health is setting limits. Boundaries are guidelines you establish to define what is acceptable or unacceptable in your relationships and interactions. Here are some practical steps for setting and maintaining boundaries for better mental health:

1. Self-Reflection:

- Reflect on your emotional needs and identify areas where you may feel overwhelmed or stressed.
- Consider past situations that led to discomfort or emotional exhaustion.

2. Identify Your Limits:

- Clearly define your emotional, physical, and time limits.
- Recognize when you start to feel uncomfortable or stressed in different situations.

3. Communicate Openly:

- Practice open communication about your needs and limits.
- Clearly express your boundaries to others in a respectful and assertive manner.

4. Be Assertive:

- Develop assertiveness in expressing your thoughts and feelings.
- Acquire the skill of saying "no" when required, guilt-free.

5. Start Small:

- Begin by setting small and manageable boundaries.
- Gradually increase the complexity as you become more comfortable.

6. Learn to Say No:

- Acknowledge that defining limits requires the ability to say "no."
- Prioritize your well-being and be firm in your decisions.

7. Understand Your Values:

- Identify your core values and use them as a guide for setting boundaries.
- Align your boundaries with what is important to you.

8. Establish Clear Consequences:

- Clearly communicate consequences for violating your boundaries.
- Be prepared to enforce consequences to maintain the integrity of your limits.

9. Trust Your Instincts:

- Trust your instincts when it comes to setting and adjusting boundaries.
- Respect your gut instinct if something doesn't seem right.

Setting boundaries is an ongoing process, and it's normal to encounter challenges along the way. By prioritizing your mental health and practicing self-awareness, you can create a framework that supports your well-being and contributes to healthier relationships.

CHAPTER EIGHT
PROFESSIONAL GUIDANCE

Seeking professional guidance is a valuable step for individuals navigating mental health challenges. Mental health professionals have the expertise to provide support, guidance, and therapeutic interventions to help individuals cope with and overcome various mental health issues. Here are key considerations and steps when seeking professional guidance:

1. Recognize the Need for Help:

- Acknowledge when you're facing challenges that impact your mental well-being.
- Understand that seeking help is a sign of strength and a proactive approach to self-care.

2. Identify the Right Professional:

- Research different mental health professionals, including psychologists, psychiatrists, counselors, and therapists.
- Consider their specialties, expertise, and the approaches they use.

3. Consult with a Primary Care Physician:

- If unsure where to start, consult with your primary care physician.
- They can provide referrals to mental health professionals and coordinate your care.

4. Understand Different Professions:

- Learn about the roles and qualifications of mental health professionals.
- For example, psychiatrists can prescribe medication, while psychologists and therapists provide counseling.

5. Consider Therapy Options:

- Explore different therapy modalities, such as cognitive-behavioral therapy (CBT), psychotherapy, or dialectical behavior therapy (DBT).
- Pick a strategy that fits your requirements and tastes.

6. Research Credentials:

- Verify the credentials and licenses of mental health professionals.
- Look for practitioners who are licensed, accredited, and have relevant experience in treating your specific concerns.

7. Read Reviews and Testimonials:

- Read reviews or testimonials from other clients to get insights into the professional's approach and effectiveness.
- Take into account asking dependable friends or family members for referrals.

8. Consider Telehealth Options:

- Explore telehealth options for remote therapy sessions, especially if in-person visits are challenging.
- Many mental health professionals offer virtual consultations.

9. Prepare for the First Appointment:

- Be prepared to discuss your concerns, symptoms, and any relevant life events during the initial appointment.
- Be open and honest to ensure an accurate assessment.

Remember that finding the right mental health professional may involve some trial and error. It's essential to prioritize your well-being and actively engage in the therapeutic process. If you encounter challenges or feel that the therapeutic relationship is not the right fit, don't hesitate to explore other options and seek a professional who aligns better with your needs.

IMPORTANCE OF SEEKING PROFESSIONAL HELP

Seeking professional help for mental health concerns is a crucial and impactful step toward overall well-being. Here are several reasons highlighting the importance of seeking professional assistance:

1. **Expertise and Specialized Knowledge:**
   - Mental health professionals, including psychologists, psychiatrists, counselors, and therapists, have specialized training and expertise in understanding and addressing various mental health issues.

2. **Accurate Diagnosis:**
   - Professionals can conduct thorough assessments to provide accurate diagnoses, which is essential for developing effective treatment plans.

3. **Individualized Treatment Plans:**
   - Mental health professionals create personalized treatment plans tailored to your specific needs, considering factors such as your symptoms, experiences, and preferences.

4. **Evidence-Based Interventions:**
   - Professionals use evidence-based interventions and therapeutic techniques that have been proven effective through research and clinical practice.

5. **Safe and Confidential Environment:**

- Therapy offers a private, secure setting where people may communicate their ideas and emotions without fear of repercussions.

6. **Emotional Support:**
   - Mental health professionals offer emotional support, empathy, and validation, helping individuals navigate their challenges.
7. **Medication Management:**
   - Psychiatrists are qualified to prescribe and manage medications when needed, providing an additional avenue for treatment.
8. **Crisis Intervention:**
   - In times of crisis or acute distress, mental health professionals can provide immediate support and intervention.
9. **Skill-Building:**
   - Therapy equips individuals with coping skills, stress management techniques, and strategies for handling challenging situations.
10. **Identification of Underlying Issues:**
    - Professionals can help identify underlying issues contributing to mental health challenges, allowing for a more comprehensive and targeted approach to treatment.

11. **Prevention of Escalation:**
    - Seeking help early can prevent the escalation of mental health issues and promote timely intervention for better outcomes.
12. **Improvement in Quality of Life:**
    - Effective mental health treatment can lead to significant improvements in overall quality of life, relationships, and daily functioning.
13. **Reduced Stigma:**
    - Normalizing seeking professional help helps reduce the stigma associated with mental health issues, fostering a more supportive and understanding society.
14. **Validation of Experiences:**
    - Mental health professionals validate individuals' experiences, acknowledging the impact of their thoughts and emotions.

15. Support for Loved Ones:
- Professionals can offer guidance and support to family members and friends, helping them understand and cope with their loved one's mental health challenges.

16. Long-Term Success:
- Professional help contributes to long-term success by addressing the root causes of mental health concerns and providing ongoing support for sustained well-being.

17. Education and Awareness:
- Mental health professionals educate individuals about their conditions, fostering self-awareness and empowering them to actively participate in their own recovery.

18. Holistic Approach:
- Professionals often take a holistic approach, addressing not only symptoms but also considering the individual's physical, social, and environmental factors.

19. Connection to Resources:
- Mental health professionals can connect individuals to additional resources, support groups, and community services that enhance their overall support network.

20. Promotion of Resilience:
- Through therapy, individuals develop resilience and adaptive coping mechanisms, enhancing their ability to navigate life's challenges.

Seeking professional help is a proactive and empowering choice that demonstrates a commitment to personal growth, well-being, and a fulfilling life. If you or someone you know is struggling with mental health concerns, reaching out to a mental health professional can be a pivotal step on the path to recovery and resilience.

THERAPY OPTIONS: COGNITIVE BEHAVIORAL THERAPY (CBT), MINDFULNESS-BASED COGNITIVE THERAPY (MBCT)

Therapy options, such as Cognitive Behavioral Therapy (CBT) and

Mindfulness-Based Cognitive Therapy (MBCT), are widely used approaches to address various mental health concerns. Each therapy has its unique principles and techniques, targeting different aspects of an individual's cognitive and emotional well-being. Here's an overview of these two therapeutic approaches:

COGNITIVE BEHAVIORAL THERAPY (CBT):

1. Overview:

- **Focus:** CBT is a goal-oriented and practical therapeutic approach that focuses on identifying and challenging negative thought patterns and behaviors.
- **Duration:** It is typically a short-term, structured therapy that involves active collaboration between the therapist and the individual.

2. Principles:

- **Cognitive Restructuring:** Individuals learn to recognize and challenge distorted or negative thought patterns and replace them with more balanced and realistic ones.
- **Behavioral Activation:** CBT often includes behavioral interventions to help individuals change unhealthy behaviors and develop healthier habits.
- **Homework Assignments:** Therapists may assign homework, such as keeping thought records or engaging in specific behavioral tasks, to reinforce learning outside of sessions.

3. Applications:

- CBT is effective in treating a wide range of mental health issues, including anxiety disorders, depression, phobias, and stress-related disorders.
- It is used in individual and group therapy settings.

4. Benefits:

- CBT provides practical tools and strategies that individuals can apply in their daily lives.
- It is structured and goal-oriented, making it suitable for addressing specific issues within a relatively short time frame.

MINDFULNESS-BASED COGNITIVE THERAPY (MBCT):

1. Overview:

- **Focus:** MBCT combines cognitive therapy with mindfulness practices to help individuals break the cycle of recurrent depressive episodes.
- **Duration:** It is often delivered in group settings and involves mindfulness training over an eight-week period.

2. Principles:

- **Mindfulness Meditation:** Individuals learn mindfulness meditation techniques to cultivate present-moment awareness, non-judgmental observation, and acceptance of thoughts and feelings.
- **Cognitive Therapy Elements:** MBCT incorporates elements of traditional CBT, particularly focusing on recognizing and changing negative thought patterns.

3. Applications:

- MBCT is specifically designed for individuals with a history of recurrent depression.
- It is also used to prevent the recurrence of depressive episodes.

4. Benefits:

- MBCT aids people in being more cognizant of their feelings and thoughts.

- It provides skills to disengage from automatic, habitual responses to negative thoughts and emotions.
- Research suggests that MBCT can be effective in preventing the recurrence of depression.

CHOOSING BETWEEN CBT AND MBCT:

1. **Nature of the Concern:**
   - CBT is versatile and can be applied to a broad range of mental health issues.
   - MBCT is specifically designed for individuals with a history of depression or those at risk of recurrent depressive episodes.

2. **Prevention vs. Treatment:**
   - CBT is widely used for both preventing and treating various mental health concerns.
   - MBCT is particularly focused on preventing the recurrence of depression.
3. **Preference for Mindfulness Practices:**
   - Individuals who are interested in mindfulness practices may find MBCT appealing.
   - CBT does not emphasize mindfulness to the same extent.
4. **Therapist's Expertise:**
   - Consider the therapist's expertise and training in each approach.
   - Some therapists may integrate elements of both CBT and mindfulness practices based on individual needs.
5. **Personal Fit:**
   - Personal preferences, comfort levels, and individual responses to each therapy approach play a crucial role in determining which one is the best fit.

It's important to note that these therapies are not mutually exclusive, and some therapists may integrate elements of both CBT and mindfulness practices based on the individual's needs. The choice between CBT and MBCT depends on the nature of the mental health concern, individual preferences, and the expertise of the therapist. Additionally, other therapeutic approaches may also be considered based on individual needs and goals. Always consult with a qualified mental health professional to determine the most appropriate therapeutic approach for your specific situation.

INTEGRATING NATURAL REMEDIES WITH PROFESSIONAL TREATMENT

Integrating natural remedies with professional treatment can be a complementary approach to support mental health. While natural remedies may offer additional benefits, it's essential to view them as supplements to, not substitutes for, evidence-based professional care. Always consult with your healthcare provider or mental health professional before incorporating natural remedies, especially if you're already receiving professional treatment. Here are some natural remedies that are commonly considered alongside professional mental health care:

1. Nutrition and Balanced Diet:

- **Importance:** Nutrition plays a crucial role in overall well-being, including mental health.
- **Tips:**
    - Consume a balanced diet with adequate nutrients, including omega-3 fatty acids, vitamins, and minerals.
    - Consider foods rich in antioxidants, such as fruits and vegetables.
    - Drink plenty of water; dehydration can impair mood and mental clarity.

2. Regular Exercise:

- **Importance:** Physical activity has been linked to improved mood, reduced stress, and enhanced cognitive function.
- **Tips:**

- Engage in regular aerobic exercise, such as walking, jogging, or swimming.
- Include strength training and flexibility exercises.
- If you want to make fitness a habit, choose something you like doing.

3. Adequate Sleep:

- **Importance:** Quality sleep is essential for mental health and overall functioning.
- **Tips:**
    - Establish a consistent sleep schedule.
    - Create a relaxing bedtime routine.
    - Ensure your sleep environment is comfortable and conducive to rest.

4. Herbal Remedies:

- **Examples:** St. John's Wort, lavender, valerian root.
- **Cautions:**
    - Consult with your healthcare provider before using herbal remedies, especially if you are taking medications.
    - Certain plants have potential negative effects or interactions with prescription drugs.

5. Mind-Body Practices:

- **Examples:** Yoga, meditation, deep breathing exercises.
- **Benefits:**
    - These practices can promote relaxation, reduce stress, and enhance mindfulness.
    - Mind-body practices are often used in conjunction with traditional therapies.

6. Aromatherapy:

- **Examples:** Essential oils like lavender, chamomile, or bergamot.

- **Methods:**
    - Use essential oils in a diffuser or apply diluted oils to pulse points.
    - Aromatherapy may contribute to a calming or uplifting atmosphere.

7. Limiting Caffeine and Sugar:

- **Importance:** Excessive caffeine and sugar intake can affect mood and energy levels.
- **Tips:**
    - Moderate your consumption of caffeinated beverages.
    - Choose whole foods over sugary snacks for stable energy levels.

8. Outdoor Activities and Nature Exposure:

- **Benefits:** Spending time in nature has been associated with improved mood and reduced stress.
- **Activities:**
    - Go for walks in parks or other natural areas..
    - Practice outdoor activities like gardening or hiking.

9. Social Support and Connections:

- **Importance:** Strong social connections contribute to mental well-being.
- **Tips:**
    - Maintain relationships with friends and family.
    - Engage in group activities or clubs to foster a sense of community.

10. Holistic Approaches:

- **Examples:** Acupuncture, massage therapy.

- **Benefits:**
    - Some individuals find these approaches helpful for relaxation and stress reduction.
    - They are often used as complementary therapies.

    Remember, natural remedies should be approached with caution and in conjunction with professional guidance. Some individuals may find these strategies beneficial, while others may not experience significant effects. Open communication with your healthcare provider ensures that any natural remedies you choose to integrate align with your overall treatment plan and do not interfere with prescribed medications or therapies.

CHAPTER NINE
SELF-CARE PRACTICES

Self-care practices are essential for maintaining and promoting mental and emotional well-being. These practices involve intentional and purposeful activities that prioritize your physical, emotional, and psychological needs. Here are various self-care practices that you can incorporate into your routine:

1. Prioritize Sleep:

- Aim for 7-9 hours of quality sleep each night.
- Make a soothing nighttime ritual and set a regular sleep regimen.

2. Regular Exercise:

- Engage in physical activity, such as walking, jogging, or yoga.
- If you want to make fitness a habit, choose something you like doing.

3. Healthy Nutrition:

- Drink enough water to stay hydrated.
- Eat a balanced diet that includes whole grains, lean meats, fruits, and vegetables.

4. Mindfulness and Meditation:

- By using mindfulness meditation, you may develop an awareness of the present moment.
- Set aside time for meditation to reduce stress and promote relaxation.

5. Deep Breathing Exercises:

- Include techniques for deep breathing to soothe the nervous system.
- Practice diaphragmatic breathing for relaxation.

6. Set Boundaries:

- Clearly state your limits and convey them to others.
- To prevent overcommitting, practice saying "no" when it's essential.

7. Digital Detox:

- Take breaks from electronic devices and social media.
- Establish designated "screen-free" periods to promote mental well-being.

8. Expressive Arts:

- Take part in artistic endeavors like writing, drawing, or performing music.
- Expressing yourself through art can be therapeutic.

9. Journaling:

- Keep a journal to explore and express your thoughts and emotions.
- Reflect on positive experiences and set goals for personal growth.

10. Quality Leisure Time:

- Make time for the things that you like and find fulfilling.

- Whether it's reading, watching a movie, or spending time in nature, prioritize leisure.

  Remember, self-care is a personal and ongoing process. It involves paying attention to your needs, acknowledging your limits, and consistently incorporating practices that contribute to your overall well-being. Regular self-care enhances resilience, reduces stress, and supports a positive and balanced lifestyle. Customize your self-care routine to align with your preferences and priorities.

MAINTAINING PROGRESS AND PREVENTING RELAPSE

Maintaining progress and preventing relapse are crucial aspects of managing mental health challenges. Here are strategies to help you sustain the positive changes you've made and reduce the risk of relapse:

1. Regular Self-Assessment:

- **Reflect:** Regularly assess your mental and emotional well-being. Pay attention to any signs of stress, anxiety, or changes in mood.
- **Track Progress:** Keep a journal or use tracking tools to monitor your progress and identify patterns.

2. Consistent Self-Care:

- **Prioritize:** Continue to prioritize self-care practices, including adequate sleep, regular exercise, and mindfulness.
- **Adapt as Needed:** Adjust your self-care routine based on changes in your life, stressors, or evolving needs.

3. Support System:

- **Stay Connected:** Maintain connections with friends, family, or support groups.
- **Open Communication:** Share your thoughts and feelings with trusted individuals. Open communication is vital for support.

4. Therapeutic Maintenance:

- **Regular Sessions:** If you're in therapy, continue attending regular sessions, even during periods of stability.
- **Adjustments:** Work with your therapist to make adjustments to your treatment plan as needed.

5. Mindfulness and Coping Skills:

- **Practice Regularly:** Continue practicing mindfulness and coping skills, especially during challenging times.
- **Integration:** Integrate these skills into your daily life to enhance resilience.

6. Set Realistic Goals:

- **Achievable Goals:** Set realistic and achievable goals. Celebrate small victories to maintain motivation.
- **Break down Tasks:** Break down larger tasks into smaller, manageable steps.

7. Identify Triggers:

- **Awareness:** Identify potential triggers for stress or negative emotions.
- **Strategies:** Develop strategies to cope with triggers and manage stress effectively.

8. Learn from Relapses:

- **Self-Reflection:** If a relapse occurs, reflect on the factors that contributed to it.

- **Learning Opportunity:** Treat relapses as learning opportunities and adjust your approach accordingly.

9. Emergency Plan:

- **Develop a Plan:** Create an emergency plan with your therapist or support system.
- **Know Resources:** Be aware of crisis helplines and emergency mental health services.

Remember that mental health is a dynamic and evolving process. Regular self-awareness, adaptive strategies, and a proactive approach to well-being contribute to maintaining progress and preventing relapse. If challenges arise, seeking professional help promptly ensures timely support and intervention.

RECOGNIZING EARLY WARNING SIGNS

Recognizing early warning signs of mental health challenges is crucial for taking proactive steps and seeking support. These signs can vary depending on the specific condition, but some general indicators may suggest that your mental health needs attention. Here are common early warning signs:

1. Changes in Mood:

- **Irritability:** Feeling easily annoyed or angered, even by small things.
- **Persistent Sadness:** Experiencing prolonged periods of low mood or sadness.

2. Sleep Disturbances:

- **Insomnia:** Difficulty falling asleep, staying asleep, or early morning awakening.
- **Excessive Sleep:** Sleeping more than usual and still feeling tired.

3. Appetite Changes:

- **Changes in Eating Habits:** Significant changes in appetite, such as overeating or loss of interest in food.

4. Energy Levels:

- **Fatigue:** Persistent lack of energy, even after adequate rest.
- **Low Motivation:** Difficulty finding motivation to engage in usual activities.

5. Difficulty Concentrating:

- **Memory Issues:** Forgetfulness and difficulty concentrating on tasks.
- **Poor Decision-Making:** Struggling with decision-making and problem-solving.

6. Social Withdrawal:

- **Isolation:** Pulling away from social activities and withdrawing from friends and family.
- **Avoidance:** Avoiding previously enjoyed social interactions.

7. Physical Symptoms:

- **Unexplained Aches and Pains:** Physical symptoms, such as headaches or stomachaches, without a clear cause.
- **Changes in Weight:** Significant weight gain or loss without intentional changes to diet or exercise.

8. Emotional Changes:

- **Heightened Anxiety:** Increased worry, tension, or restlessness.
- **Emotional Sensitivity:** Heightened sensitivity to criticism or perceived slights.

9. Changes in Performance:

- **Work or Academic Decline:** A noticeable decline in performance at work or school.
- **Decreased Productivity:** Difficulty completing tasks that were once manageable.

If you or someone you know is experiencing multiple signs of distress, seeking professional help is crucial. Mental health professionals can provide support, assessment, and guidance for appropriate intervention. Early recognition and intervention often lead to better outcomes in managing mental health challenges.

IMPORTANCE OF REGULAR CHECK-INS WITH PROFESSIONALS

Regular check-ins with mental health professionals are crucial for several reasons, and they play a significant role in maintaining and improving mental well-being. Here are some key reasons highlighting the importance of regular check-ins with mental health professionals:

1. Monitoring Progress:

- **Assessment:** Professionals can assess your progress in managing mental health challenges.
- **Adjustments:** Regular check-ins allow for adjustments to treatment plans based on your evolving needs.

2. Early Intervention:

- **Identification of Issues:** Professionals can identify early signs of relapse or emerging challenges.

- **Preventive Measures:** Early intervention can prevent issues from escalating and improve long-term outcomes.

3. Medication Management:

- **Effectiveness:** For individuals on medication, regular check-ins ensure that medications are effective.
- **Adjustments:** Professionals can make necessary adjustments to dosage or medication type based on your response.

4. Therapeutic Relationship:

- **Trust and Rapport:** Regular check-ins contribute to the development of trust and rapport with your therapist or mental health provider.
- **Communication:** A strong therapeutic relationship fosters open communication about your experiences and concerns.

5. Support System:

- **Emotional Support:** Professionals provide a consistent source of emotional support.
- **Validation:** Validation of your experiences and emotions contributes to a sense of understanding.

6. Skill Building:

- **Skill Development:** Check-ins provide opportunities to reinforce and build upon coping skills.
- **Learning:** Professionals can introduce new strategies for managing challenges and enhancing resilience.

7. Preventing Isolation:

- **Reducing Isolation:** Regular interactions with professionals reduce feelings of isolation.

- **Connection:** The therapeutic relationship provides a valuable connection for individuals who may feel socially isolated.

8. Continuity of Care:

- **Consistency:** Regular check-ins contributes to the continuity of care.
- **Comprehensive Approach:** Professionals can take a comprehensive approach to address multiple aspects of mental health.

9. Monitoring Side Effects:

- **Medication Side Effects:** For those on medication, professionals can monitor and address any potential side effects.
- **Holistic Health:** Check-ins considers the holistic impact of treatments on overall well-being.

> Regular check-ins creates a consistent and supportive framework for individuals navigating mental health challenges. They contribute to ongoing care, prevention, and the promotion of overall well-being. The frequency of check-ins may vary depending on individual needs, treatment plans, and the nature of mental health conditions. Always communicate openly with your mental health provider about your preferences and concerns.

CHAPTER TEN
CONCLUSION

In conclusion, addressing and managing depression involves a multifaceted approach that considers biological, psychological, social, and lifestyle factors. The integration of natural remedies, mind-body practices, social support, and professional guidance creates a comprehensive strategy for mental well-being. Here are key takeaways:

1. Holistic Understanding:

- **Biological Factors:** Biological aspects, including genetics and neurochemistry, contribute to depression.
- **Psychological Factors:** Cognitive patterns, thought processes, and emotional experiences influence mental health.
- **Social Factors:** Social connections, relationships, and societal influences impact well-being.

2. Lifestyle Changes:

- **Diet and Nutrition:** A balanced diet supports overall health, including mental well-being.
- **Regular Exercise:** Physical activity has a positive impact on mood and can be a powerful tool in managing depression.
- **Adequate Sleep:** Quality sleep is crucial for mental health, and sleep hygiene practices contribute to well-being.

3. Natural Remedies:

- **Herbal Remedies:** Certain herbs, such as St. John's Wort, lavender oil, and valerian root, may offer calming effects.
- **Mind-Body Practices:** Practices like yoga, meditation, and deep breathing exercises contribute to mental well-being.
- **Holistic Approaches:** Acupuncture, massage therapy, and aromatherapy provide additional avenues for emotional balance.

4. Social Support and Connections:

- **Building a Support System:** Cultivate diverse connections and engage in supportive relationships.
- **Positive Relationships:** Positive connections contribute to emotional support and reduce feelings of isolation.
- **Joining Supportive Communities:** Online and local communities provide shared experiences and a sense of belonging.

5. Limiting Negative Influences:

- **Managing Social Media and Screen Time:** Set boundaries to prevent negative impacts on mental health.
- **Recognizing and Avoiding Toxic Relationships:** Establish clear boundaries and seek positive connections.
- **Setting Boundaries for Mental Health:** Prioritize self-care by setting and maintaining boundaries.

6. Professional Guidance:

- **Importance of Seeking Professional Help:** Early intervention and personalized treatment plans are crucial.
- **Therapy Options:** Cognitive Behavioral Therapy (CBT), Mindfulness-Based Cognitive Therapy (MBCT), and medication are effective interventions.
- **Integrating Natural Remedies with Professional Treatment:** Collaboration with healthcare providers ensures a comprehensive and safe approach.

7. Self-Care Practices:

- **Establishing a Self-Care Routine:** Consistent self-care, including sleep, exercise, and relaxation, contributes to overall well-being.
- **Maintaining Progress and Preventing Relapse:** Regular self-assessment, mindfulness, and adapting to changing needs are key to sustained progress.

8. Recognizing Early Warning Signs:

- **Changes in Mood, Sleep, and Appetite:** Pay attention to shifts in emotional and physical well-being.
- **Social Withdrawal and Changes in Behavior:** Notice signs of isolation or avoidance of once-enjoyed activities.
- **Seeking Professional Help Promptly:** Addressing early warning signs promptly contributes to better outcomes.

9. Continuation of Natural Remedies:

- **Herbal Remedies (Continued):** Valerian root, passionflower, and kava are additional options with calming effects.
- **Mind-Body Practices (Continued):** Yoga, various meditation techniques, and deep breathing exercises provide ongoing benefits.
- **Holistic Approaches (Continued):** Acupuncture, massage therapy, and aromatherapy continue to support emotional well-being.

10. Conclusion:

- **Comprehensive Approach:** Depression management involves a combination of lifestyle changes, natural remedies, social support, and professional guidance.
- **Individualized Care:** Tailoring interventions to individual needs promotes a holistic and effective approach.
- **Ongoing Self-Care:** Regular check-ins with professionals, self-assessment, and adapting strategies contribute to sustained well-being.

Remember, the journey to managing depression is unique for each individual, and seeking professional guidance is a crucial step. Integrating various strategies and staying attuned to personal needs can contribute to a more comprehensive and effective approach to mental well-being.